Computers in Health Care

Kathryn J. Hannah   Marion J. Ball
Series Editors

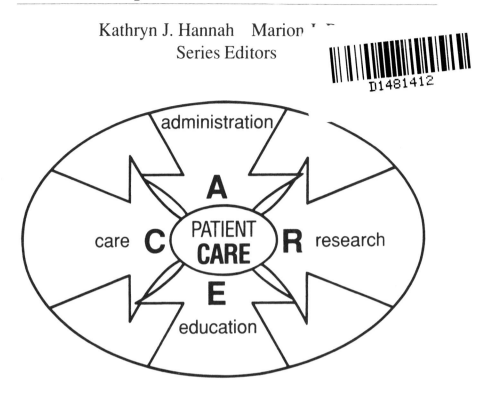

Springer

New York
Berlin
Heidelberg
Barcelona
Hong Kong
London
Milan
Paris
Singapore
Tokyo

Health Informatics Series
(formerly Computers in Health Care)

Series Editors
Kathryn J. Hannah   Marion J. Ball

Dental Informatics
Integrating Technology into the Dental Environment
L.M. Abbey and J. Zimmerman

Aspects of the Computer-based Patient Record
M.J. Ball and M.F. Collen

Performance Improvement Through Information Management
Health Care's Bridge to Success
M.J. Ball and J.V. Douglas

Strategies and Technologies for Healthcare Information
Theory into Practice
M.J. Ball, J.V. Douglas, and D.E. Garets

Nursing Informatics
Where Caring and Technology Meet, Second Edition
M.J. Ball, K.J. Hannah, S.K. Newbold, and J.V. Douglas

Healthcare Information Management Systems
A Practical Guide, Second Edition
M.J. Ball, D.W. Simborg, J.W. Albright, and J.V. Douglas

Clinical Decision Support Systems
Theory and Practice
E.S. Berner

Strategy and Architecture of Health Care Information Systems
M.K. Bourke

Information Networks for Community Health
P.F. Brennan, S.J. Schneider, and E. Tornquist

Introduction to Clinical Informatics
P. Degoulet and M. Fieschi

Patient Care Information Systems
Successful Design and Implementation
E.L. Drazen, J.B. Metzger, J.L. Ritter, and M.K. Schneider

Introduction to Nursing Informatics, Second Edition
K.J. Hannah, M.J. Ball, and M.J.A. Edwards

Computerizing Large Integrated Health Networks
The VA Success
R.M. Kolodner

Organizational Aspects of Health Informatics
Managing Technological Change
N.M. Lorenzi and R.T. Riley

(continued after Index)

Patrice Degoulet   Marius Fieschi

Introduction to
Clinical Informatics

Benjamin Phister
Translator

With 157 Illustrations

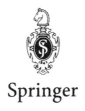

Springer

Patrice Degoulet
Professeur
Faculté de Médecine
Broussais Hôtel-Dieu
Université Pierre et Marie Curie
96 rue Didot
75014 Paris, France

Marius Fieschi
Professeur
Faculté de Médecine
Université d'Aix – Marseille II
254 rue Saint-Pierre
13385 Marseille, France

Library of Congress Cataloging-in-Publication Data
Degoulet, Patrice.
   [Informatique medicale. English]
   Introduction to Clinical Informatics / Patrice Degoulet, Marius Fieschi.
     p.   cm. – (Computers in health care)
   Includes bibliographical references and index.
   ISBN 0-387-94641-1 (hardcover:alk. paper)
   1. Medicine – Data processing.   2. Medical care – Data processing.
  I. Fieschi, M. (Marius) II. Title. III. Series.
  R858.D434   1996
  362.1′0285 – dc20   96-18687

Printed on acid-free paper.

Production managed by Hal Henglein; manufacturing supervised by Joe Quatela.
Camera-ready copy supplied by the authors.
Printed and bound by Maple-Vail Book Manufacturing Group, York, PA.
Printed in the United States of America.

9 8 7 6 5 4 3 2 (Corrected second printing, 1999)

ISBN 0-387-94641-1 Springer-Verlag New York Berlin Heidelberg   SPIN 10730429

To François Grémy

Foreword

Introduction to Clinical Informatics fills a void in the Computer in Health Care series. With this volume, Patrice Degoulet and Marius Fieschi provide a comprehensive view of medical informatics and carry that concept forward into the realm of clinical informatics. The authors draw upon their experiences as medical school faculty members in France, where informatics has long been integrated into the curriculum and where the French version of this very book has been used, tested, and revised.

In intent and content, this volume stands as the companion volume to Introduction to Nursing Informatics, one of the series' best selling titles. For practitioners and students of medicine, pharmacy, and other health professions, Introduction to Clinical Informatics offers an essential understanding how computing can support patient care, clarifying practical uses and critical issues.

Today medical schools in the United States are making informatics a part of their curriculum, with required medical informatics blocks at the onset of training serving as the base for problem-based learning throughout the course of study. In an increasingly networked and computerized environment, health-care providers are having to alter how they practice. Whether in the office, the clinic, or the hospital, health-care professionals have access to a growing array of capabilities and tools as they deliver care. Learning to use these becomes a top priority, and this volume becomes a valuable resource.

As medical informaticians, Degoulet and Fieschi devote several chapters to the nature of medical information, including medical data, medical reasoning, and medical language. All too often slighted, these concepts are key to understanding the applications of computers in medicine, from knowledge databases to medical decision making and more. The authors also address critical concerns regarding the analysis and control of medical activity and the security and protection of medical data. These are issues which we must confront if we are to make optimal use of the technologies available to us.

The authors have chosen to dedicate this volume to Francois Grémy, who founded the discipline of medical informatics in France and who served as the first president of the International Medical Informatics Association (IMIA). It is a worthy tribute. As one of those honored to follow Francois as IMIA president, I take pride in endorsing this volume. It represents the discipline which IMIA has sponsored and bodes well for IMIA's future. Patrice Degoulet has served as cochair of the scientific program committee for the ninth triennial IMIA congress, known as MedInfo, held in Korea in 1998.

In their preface, Degoulet and Fieschi call this work "a snapshot of the equilibrium between methodology and applications of computers in medicine at a given moment in time, based on constantly changing technologies." It is that and it is more. It truly embodies the discipline as it is and as it will evolve.

What was theory is now becoming practice. The vision we nurtured in IMIA is now beginning to nurture us, as professionals and as patients. What began as medical informatics and matured as health informatics is now truly evolving into clinical informatics.

To Patrice and Marius, our thanks for carrying on the IMIA tradition. For those young health care informaticians and practitioners who will take the discipline into the next century, the Introduction to Clinical Informatics will be an invaluable guide.

Marion J. Ball

Series Preface

This series is intended for the rapidly increasing number of health care professionals who have rudimentary knowledge and experience in health care computing and are seeking opportunities to expand their horizons. It does not attempt to compete with the primers already on the market. Eminent international experts will edit, author, or contribute to each volume in order to provide comprehensive and current accounts of innovation and future trends in this quickly evolving field. Each book will be practical, easy to use and well referenced.

Our aim is for the series to encompass all of the health professions by focusing on specific professions, such as nursing, in individual volumes. However, integrated computing systems are only one tool for improving communication among members of the health care team. Therefore, it is our hope that the series will stimulate professionals to explore additional means of fostering interdisciplinary exchange.

This series springs from a professional collaboration that has grown over the years into a highly valued personal friendship. Our joint values put people first. If the Computers in Health Care series lets us share those values by helping health care professionals to communicate their ideas for the benefit of patients, than our efforts will have succeeded.

Kathryn J. Hannah
Marion J. Ball

Preface

If a group of doctors, computer scientists, or scientists from other disciplines were asked the question "What is medical informatics?", the response would certainly not be unanimous. Some might point out concrete examples, viewing applications in the area of medical computing as a set of techniques and tools. Others would emphasize the technology itself, its progress in recent years, or its future perspectives. These replies describe the tip of the iceberg, since they present medical computing only through its applications and techniques. This is due to the rather peculiar development of computing, which is driven by technical developments: "Technical capabilities came first, founded as always on a science, solid physics, but a stranger to its own subject, information processing" [Arsac 1983].

Medical informatics is also a scientific discipline. It helps us to understand the mechanics of medical interpretation and medical reasoning, of the abstraction and elaboration of knowledge, and of memorization and learning. The science of managing medical information is at the very foundation of medicine. What is medical information? What is the process that lets us go from symptom to diagnosis and then to decision? What is the validity of a decision-making strategy? What are the mechanisms of medical discovery? Can we define an ethics of information processing? These are a few of the questions to which medical informatics may provide possible answers. Like other scientific disciplines, it includes a cultural and sociological dimension that gives it a special place among basic medical disciplines.

Medical informatics helps us to gather and record facts, but also to interpret them. It provides knowledge about knowledge and, therefore, concerns all areas of medicine, from the microscopic to the macroscopic, and from individual care to public health.

Medical informatics is a science that, like other disciplines such as molecular biology or the neurosciences, has it roots in the history and ideas of information theory. It is characterized by its subject (medicine) and its methods (those of information management). Medical informatics calls upon other disciplines such as mathematics, statistics, linguistics and the science of cognition or philosophy. It is well suited to an experimental approach: suggestion of a hypothesis; modeling; experimentation, often in the form of the development or implementation of programs or prototypes of information systems; evaluation; validation; and, eventually, generalization of the process.

Modern, quality-oriented medicine requires the rational management of medical information. As medicine increases in complexity (due to new methods of investigation or treatment and the diversification of health-care organizations), medical informatics is an indispensable agent for federation and integration. It helps to overcome human limitations in memorizing or processing information (e.g., managing complex medical objects such as signals or images, reconstructing images, optimizing the dosage of certain medications, managing large bases of medical knowledge). By implementing communication networks, it helps bring the physician closer to the patient (e.g., through telemedicine) and facilitates access to information required for optimal care (e.g., through access to knowledge bases, the use of expert systems, or cooperative work).

Clinical informatics is the subset of medical informatics that is mainly concerned with clinical practice. In some extent, it represents for medical informatics what clinical epidemiology is for epidemiology.

This book is an introduction to clinical informatics. It is designed not only for students of medicine, pharmacy, and dentistry, but also for practicing physicians and health-care professionals who need an overview of the issues as well as the practical uses of computing in health care. It does not require any specialized mathematical or statistical knowledge.

The first two chapters cover the hardware and software tools for medical information processing and familiarize the reader with computing terminology and methodology. The next three chapters concern medical information, the object of medical informatics. They discuss the problems of the nature of medical data and semiology (Chapter 3), medical reasoning and decision-making (Chapter 4), and the language of medicine as a vehicle for data and knowledge (Chapter 5).

Chapters 6 through 13 illustrate the various applications of clinical informatics through concrete examples: information and knowledge databases (Chapter 6), hospital information systems (Chapter 7), health-care networks and computerized health information systems (Chapter 9), signal and image processing (Chapters 10 and 11), medical decision support systems (Chapter 12), and computer-based education (Chapter 13).

The last two chapters concern two particular aspects of clinical informatics. As an architecture for gathering and processing medical information, clinical informatics may help measure and evaluate medical activity (Chapter 14). Chapter 15 calls for reflection on the limitations and dangers of computerized medicine and defines appropriate measures to reconcile respect for individual liberties and the benefits computerized medicine brings to the individual as well as the community.

Reviews of probabilities and logic are provided in the appendices. The principal technical terms used in computing and their definitions may be found in the glossary.

This work represents a snapshot of computer methodology and applications in medicine at a given moment in time, while the technology is constantly changing. It is dedicated to François Grémy, the founder of the discipline in France and the first president of the International Medical Informatics Association (IMIA). A number of people have provided comments and criticism, and we would particularly like to thank Françoise Aimé, Geneviève Botti, Gilles Chatellier, Pierre Corvol, Dominique Fieschi, Isabelle Fofol, Didier Heudes, François-Christophe Jean, Joanny Gouvernet, Marie-Christine Jaulent, Michel Joubert, Eric Lepage, Joël Ménard, Isabelle Perré, Dominique Sauquet, and Gérard Soula.

When we were preparing a revised version of the French edition of this textbook, Marion Ball and Kathryn Hannah greatly encouraged us to prepare simultaneously an English version. Benjamin Phister made this possible by translating each chapter as soon as it was ready. We are indebted to them for their warm and constant support.

Patrice Degoulet
Marius Fieschi

Contents

Foreword   vi

Series Preface   viii

Preface   ix

Chapter 1. Systems for Managing Medical Information   1

Introduction 1
Principles of Computer Operations 1
Hardware Architecture 2
    Encoding Information in a Machine 2
    The Memory Hierarchy 3
    Computer Categories 5
    Central Processing Unit Operations 7
    Input-Output Peripherals 7
Software Architecture 8
    Operating Systems 8
    Development Environments and Utilities 9
    Application Programs 11
Communications and Networks 12
    Network Architecture 12
    Standards for Exchanging Information 13
Integrated System Architectures 14
    Centralized Systems 14
    Distributed Systems 15
    Multimedia Workstations 16
    Network of Networks 16
Exercises 17

Chapter 2. Medical Software Development   19

Introduction 19
Computer Project Management 19
    Waterfall Models 19
    Spiral Methods and Quick Prototyping 22
Conceptual Models 23
    The Notion of a Model 23
    Objects and Relationships 24
    Modeling Intermediate Structures 24
    Semantic Networks 25
Software Development Tools 26
    Computer-Aided Software Engineering 26
    Database Management Systems 27
    Document Management Systems 31

Interface Management Systems 32
Natural Language Processing Tools 32
Specialized Software Components 32
Electronic Data Interchange 33
Integrating Software Components 33
Exercises 34

Chapter 3. Medical Data and Semiology   35

Introduction 35
The Nature of Medical Data 36
Medical Data Types 36
The Variability of Medical Data 36
Interpreting Medical Data 38
Cognitive Processes 38
Interpreting Numbers and Words 38
Interpreting Associations 39
Quantitative Semiology 39
The Diagnostic Value of a Test 39
Sensitivity and Specificity of a Sign 41
Measuring the Predictive Value of a Sign 44
Discussion and Conclusions 46
Exercises 47

Chapter 4. Medical Reasoning and Decision-Making   49

Introduction 49
Reasoning 49
Deduction 49
Induction 50
Abduction 50
Causal Reasoning 51
The Steps Involved in Making a Medical Decision 51
Identify the Problem 52
Structure the Problem 52
Choose the Solution 52
Uncertainty and Medical Judgment 53
Medical Judgment 53
Uncertainty and Judgment Bias 53
Probability Theory and Decision Analysis 54
Comparing Several Diagnostic Hypotheses 54
Evaluating the Benefits of Therapy 55
Decision Analysis 57
Symbolic Reasoning and Expert Systems 58
Knowledge Representation 59
Using Knowledge 60
Learning 63
Discussion and Conclusion 64

Exercises 64

Chapter 5. Medical Language and Classification Systems 65

Introduction 65
Coding and Classifications 65
Examples of Classifications 68
    Clinical Classifications 68
    The NANDA Classification of Nursing Diagnoses 71
    Classification of Treatments and Procedures 71
    Multidomain Classifications 73
Discussion and Conclusion 79
Exercises 80

Chapter 6. Documentation Systems and Information Databases 81

Introduction 81
Technical Infrastructure 81
    Workstations 81
    Connecting to Networks 82
    Archiving and Server Functions 82
General Characteristics 82
    Document Mediation 82
    The Quality of a Documentation Management System 83
Documentation Systems 84
    Bibliographical Databases 84
    Medical Information and Knowledge Bases 86
Discussion and Conclusion 88
Exercises 89

Chapter 7. Hospital Information Systems 91

Introduction 91
Analysis of the Information System 92
    The Various Levels of the Information System 92
    The Environment of the Information System 92
    HIS Objectives 93
    Structural Analysis 94
    Functional Analysis 95
The Components of an HIS 96
    Administration 96
    Health-Care Units 96
    Ancillary Departments 97
Strategies and Technical Solutions 98
    The Vertical Approach: Centralized HIS 98
    The Horizontal Approach: Departmental Systems 100
    The Distributed Approach: Distributed and Open Systems 100

Required Resources 102
    Allocating Resources and Estimating Costs 102
    Human Resources 103
Discussion and Conclusion 103
Exercises 104

Chapter 8. Health-Care Networks   105

Introduction 105
The Health System 106
    Health-Care Coverage 106
    Medical Demographics 107
Health-Care Networks and Health Information Systems 109
    The Components of a Health-Care Network 109
    Telemedicine Tools in Health-Care Networks 110
    Data Access and Communications 111
The Information System for Generalists 112
    The Key Role of the Generalist in the Health-Care Network 112
    Computerizing the Doctor's Office 113
The Patient's Information System 114
    Active Participation in Health Care 115
    Training at Home 115
    Electronic Messaging 115
Discussion and Conclusion 115
Exercises 116

Chapter 9. Managing Patient Records   117

Introduction 117
Different Views of Patient Records 118
Objectives and Expected Benefits 119
Modeling Medical Information 121
    How to Standardize Medical Terminology 122
    How to Structure Medical Records 122
Implementing Computerized Medical Records 126
    The Software Environment 126
    Patient Management Systems 128
    Hardware and Human Constraints 129
Discussion and Conclusion 130
Exercises 130

Chapter 10. Physiological Signal Processing   131

Introduction 131
Importance and Objectives 131
Basic Signal Processing Concepts 132
    Signal Acquisition 132
    Sampling and Digitizing Signals 132
    Basic Signal Processing Techniques 133

Sample Medical Applications 135
    Examples of Signal Analysis 135
    Intensive Care Monitoring 136
    Integration in Information Systems 137
Discussion and Conclusion 137
Exercises 138

Chapter 11. Medical Imaging Systems   139

Introduction 139
Importance and Objectives 139
Image Acquisition Sources 140
Digitized Images 142
    Spatial Coding 142
    Intensity Coding 143
    Temporal Coding 143
    Digitizing Images 143
Basic Image Processing Principles 144
    The Imaging Process 144
    Image Preprocessing 145
    Segmentation 146
    Extracting Parameters 146
    Image Interpretation 147
Sample Medical Applications 147
    Quantifying the Degree of a Vascular Stenosis 147
    Identifying Chromosomes 147
    Computer-Aided Surgical Techniques 148
    Virtual Reality 149
Imaging Management and Communication Systems 150
    Tele-expertise 150
    PACS 150
Discussion and Conclusion 151
Exercises 152

Chapter 12. Medical Decision Support Systems   153

Introduction 153
Characteristics of Decision Support Systems 154
    Types of Support 154
    Types of Intervention 154
    Types of Knowledge 155
Methodological Basis of Decision Support Systems 156
    Using Mathematical Models 156
    Statistical Methods 156
    Probability-Based Systems 157
    Artificial Intelligence and Expert Systems 158
    Neural Networks and Connectionist Systems 159
Implementing Decision Support Systems 160

The User Interface 161
Knowledge Acquisition and Representation 161
Evaluating and Validating Systems 161
Integrating Decision Support Modules in Information Systems .. 162
Sample Decision Support Systems 162
Pharmacokinetics and Assistance in Calculating Dosages 162
Assistance in Diagnosing Acute Abdominal Pain 163
Diagnoses in Internal Medicine: INTERNIST and QMR 163
Assistance in Chemotherapy: ONCOCIN 164
Integration in a Hospital Information System: HELP 164
Decision Support in Molecular Biology 165
Discussion and Conclusion 166
Exercises 167

Chapter 13. Computer-Based Education — 169

Introduction 169
The Need for a Global Pedagogical Approach 169
The Role of Computer-Based Education 171
Methods and Implementations 172
Tutorial Training 172
Modeling and Simulation 174
On-Site Teaching 175
Intelligent CBE Systems 176
Discussion and Conclusion 177
Exercises 178

Chapter 14. Analysis and Control of Medical Activity — 179

Introduction 179
Controlling Health-Care Expenses 179
Evaluation, Control, and Quality 180
Methods and Principles for Analyzing Medical Activity 182
A General Model 182
Evaluating Costs 182
Two Approaches for "Medicalized" Management 183
Analyzing Medical Activity in the Hospital 184
Resource Indicators 184
Activity Indicators 184
Production Indicators 185
Quality Indicators 191
Discussion and Conclusion 192
Exercises 192

Chapter 15. Security and Data Protection — 193

Introduction 193
Identifying the Risks 193
Protecting Data Concerning Individuals 194

Professional Ethics and Legal Measures 194
Measures Concerning Hardware, Software, and Organization ... 198
Discussion and Conclusion 200
Exercises 200

Appendix A. Review of Probabilities   201

Introduction 201
Conditional Probabilities 201
Bayes' Formula 202
Relative Risk and Odds Ratio 202

Appendix B. Review of Logic   205

Introduction 205
Propositional Logic 205
Predicate Logic 207

Appendix C. Some Useful References   209

Medical Informatics Associations 209
In France 209
In Europe 209
In the United States 209
The International Medical Informatics Association 210
Principal International Conferences 210
Principal Specialized Publications 210
Internet Addresses 211
General Catalogs and Electronic Libraries 211
Informatics in Health Care and Telemedicine, Standards 211
Medical Informatics Textbooks 211
Data and Knowledge Banks 212
Medical guidelines, Evidence-Based Medicine 212

Bibliography   213

Glossary   225

Index   231

1

Systems for Managing Medical Information

Introduction

Informatics, the science of information management, employs a variety of techniques to automate the collection, storage, utilization, and transmission of information. Because it relies on the use of computers, informatics requires that information be represented in an encoded, computer-readable format.

The first computer applications were limited to numerical calculations and simple administrative tasks. In the last decade, computers have evolved to manage more and more complex elements such as images and sounds, often referred to as *multimedia objects*. At the same time, the development of communication networks has enabled the interconnection of computer systems, allowing previously independent applications to interact. Today enterprises are able to build their information systems from computers, networks, and communication protocols much like an urban architect plans and builds a new city.

This chapter provides a succinct review of the techniques used in medical information systems. It is organized around the following themes: the hardware and software fundamentals of computing; methods for encoding information so that it can be processed by computers; communications networks; and hardware and software architectures for information systems.

Principles of Computer Operations

Computers process information that has been stored in their central memory according to a predefined sequence of instructions called a *computer program*. Programs are written in a language that the machine can understand called a *programming language*. Figure 1.1 illustrates basic computer architecture.

The *central processing unit* (CPU), or processor, executes the instructions contained in the program according to the logical sequence or algorithm determined by the programmer. Operations are performed on the data provided as input to the program, which then calculates the results, called output. The processor and central memory make up the central processing unit of the computer. They communicate over an internal electronic circuit called the communication bus. The central processor is usually composed of an arithmetic-logic unit (ALU), which performs the calculations, and a control unit, which manages the execution sequence of the program instructions.

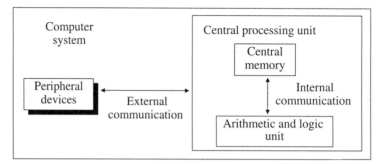

Figure 1.1 : Basic principles of data processing systems

Input and output data coexist with the program in the computer's central memory. Input data and programs are transmitted to the central processing unit via the input peripherals. Results coming from the central processing unit may be stored on output peripherals.

Hardware Architecture

The fundamental architecture of the majority of modern computers is a more- or less-sophisticated version of the Von Neumann architecture presented in figure 1.1. Differences include the modalities of coding information in the machine, memory organization, performance, and the number of processors used (Figure 1.2).

Encoding Information in a Machine

All data are represented by a combination of items called binary digits, or *bits*. Electronics makes possible the construction of elements that are stable in either of two states, conventionally called "0" and "1". Bit sequences are used to represent both the program instructions and the data manipulated by the programs (numbers, alphabetic characters, images, sounds, etc.). Two bits may encode four states (00, 01, 10, and 11), three bits encode eight states, and so on. A group of eight bits is a *byte*, and can represent one of 256 possible combinations. This is sufficient to encode the principal typographical characters of an Indo-European language. Figure 1.3 illustrates the principle of binary representation for an integer in one byte.

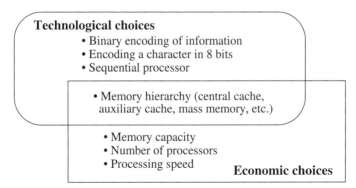

Figure 1.2 : Data processing strategies

The ASCII code (American Standard Code for Information Interchange) is a seven-bit standard code representing 128 characters, while the ISO (International Standards Organization) Latin-1 code is an extension of the ASCII code to eight bits. Text may thus be encoded as of a set of bytes. Other conventions have been established to represent numbers or more complex objects such as images. Unfortunately, these may vary from one computer to another, often requiring special transcoding programs. The characters on a Macintosh computer, for example, are encoded differently from those on an IBM PC.

Decimal	Binary	Power of
0	0	
1	1	
2	10	2
3	11	
4	100	2^2
5	101	
6	110	
7	111	
8	1000	2^3

Representation of the number 90
in one byte

$64 + 16 + 8 + 2 = 90$
$2^6 \quad 2^4 \ 2^3 \quad 2^1$

0	1	0	1	1	0	1	0
7	6	5	4	3	2	1	0

Position of the binary
digit in the byte

Figure 1.3 : The binary representation of an integer in one byte

Program instructions are normally encoded in memory in a small number of bytes (e.g., 2, 3, 4, or 8), creating "words" of 16, 24, 32, or 64 bits.

The Memory Hierarchy

Computers utilize many types of memory differentiated by their access time, capacity, and unit cost. Memory size is expressed in kilobytes (K), megabytes (MB) and gigabytes (GB). In order to optimize the price/performance characteristics of a given system, memory is usually organized in hierarchical levels (Figure 1.4).

Central Processing Unit Memory

CPU memory is characterized by high cost per byte and short access times (under one microsecond). This is *direct access* memory, meaning the contents of a single byte or word may be addressed at a given time. This memory is usually volatile: the contents are lost when the computer is turned off.

Three main types of memory may be distinguished:

- *Registers* are regions of memory in the arithmetic-logic unit in which elementary operations (e.g., addition, subtraction, or multiplication) may be performed very rapidly. The number of registers is limited.
- *Cache memory* is used to accelerate transfers between processors and central memory.
- *Central memory* is the base memory of the CPU, containing both data and instructions. Each byte or word in central memory may be addressed directly, in any order. It is often called *random access memory* (RAM). Central memory may be accessed in a set time, on the order of a few nanoseconds.

Type of Memory	Access time	Size
CPU memory		
- Register	0.1 – 10 ns	8 –32 registers
- Cache memory	10 – 50 ns	32 K– 1 MB
- Central memory	10 – 500 ns	32 MB – 16 GB
Peripheral memory		
- Magnetic disks	5 – 100 ms	100 MB – 20 GB
- Optical disks	100 – 300 ms	650 MB – 18 GB
- Magnetic tapes	100 – 2000 s	100 MB – 24 GB
- Microprocessor-based cards	1 – 5 ms	16 K– 256 K

Figure 1.4 : Memory hierarchy

Peripheral Memory

Peripheral memory is characterized by low cost per byte, high capacity (hence the name *mass memory*), and longer access times, from a few microseconds to a few seconds. Some peripheral memory is removable and may be used for backup copies of data. This memory is not addressed by byte or by word but by groups of bytes of a given length called *blocks*. Capacity ranges from several kilobytes up to several gigabytes, which are required for the storage of some multimedia documents. For example, a high-definition color image may occupy a few hundred kilobytes. A 6-minute video sequence, once digitized, requires approximately 2 MB in normal definition and up to ten times more in high definition.

Peripheral memory comes in many categories:

- *Removable magnetic diskettes* store from 1 to 2 MB on a diskette 3.5 in. (9 cm) in diameter. For example, a single high-density diskette of 1.4 MB contains the equivalent of 300 typewritten pages.

- *Magnetic hard disks*, either fixed or removable, have capacities that range from a few dozen megabytes to a few gigabytes. Swapping zones may be reserved on certain hard disks to accelerate the exchange of data from central memory to peripheral memory and to save all or some of the data contained in central memory.

- *Removable optical numerical disks* are available as CD-ROM (compact disc - read-only memory), WORM (write once-read many) or WMRM (write many-read many). The most common size for the first generation of CD-ROMs, WORMs, and WMRM is 5.25 in.(13 cm) for a capacity of approximately 650 MB (or the equivalent of 250,000 pages of text). The most frequently used storage protocol is ISO 9660. Audio compact discs (CD-audio) and interactive compact discs (CD-I) use a different storage format. The second generation is a high-density 5.25 in. format (DVD, for *Digital Versatile Disk*) that is able to store from 4.7 GB to 18 GB of data (the equivalent of 2 to 6 hours of compressed video) and will unify the storage format for these different data types.

- *Memory cards* quickly became popular following the development of banking cards. They are a plastic medium in a standard size (8.5 x 5.4 cm), and one or several magnetic strips are affixed to the back. A relatively small amount of information is stored on the card: approximately 200 characters for a bank card. The addition of a microprocessor transforms the card into a more intelligent device for storing information (an actual peripheral memory) and also a system for access control and processing (a real computer). The capacity of a microprocessor-based card (*smart card*) ranges from 16 to 256 K. It is possible to define parts of the memory that cannot be overwritten (EPROM technology, for electrically programmable read-only memory) and parts that can be erased (EEPROM, for electrically erasable programmable read-only memory). The intelligence feature of the card is particularly interesting for security functions, such as the identification and authentication of the user, the first step to controlling access to an information system.

Computer Categories

Most computers are based on high-performance, integrated microprocessors, such as the Motorola 68xxx, the Intel 80x86, the SUN Sparc, or the Compaq/ Digital Equipment Corporation Alpha. Improvements in computer performance, memory and communication components allows a 30% to 50% annual improvement in the price/performance ratio of computer systems, while their physical size decreases.

Six major computer categories may be distinguished, although performance criteria are becoming increasingly relative:

- *Mainframe computers* allow a large number of users (hundreds) to connect to and share large processing resources.

- *Minicomputers* were introduced in the 1960s to meet the needs of small groups of users (a few dozen) or to be dedicated to a particular task such as the management of a biological analysis laboratory.

- *Microcomputers*, corresponding to the concept of personal or individual computers (PCs), appeared in the 1970s following the commercial availability of the microprocessor. These systems made possible the development of *intelligent terminals*, capable of local processing (e.g., graphics) and *workstations*. The architecture of workstations is indistinguishable from that of other computers (Figure 1.5).

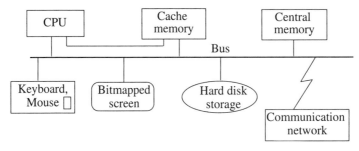

Figure 1.5 : Typical microcomputer architecture

- *Portable microcomputers* are nearly the size of an 8.5 x 11 in. sheet of paper (hence the name *notebook*). They weigh between 1 and 3 kg, offer from 2 to 6 hours of autonomy, and may be connected to networks directly, via modem, or via wireless connections using infrared or radio waves.

- *Hand-held computers* or *personal digital assistants* (PDAs) are small enough to be carried around in a coat pocket or a handbag. Their use is likely to become more widespread with improvements in handwriting recognition software and wireless communications facilities (via infrared or Hertzian techniques), which will allow the mobile entry or consultation of data on computer notepads and synchronization with desktop computers (e.g., electronic mails, contacts, to do lists).

- *Network computers* (NCs) are low-cost microcomputers developed for easing access to networks such as the Internet. They extend the Minitel concept developed in France in the early 1970s (currently installed in more than 10 million locations). Peripheral memory is not necessary since data files can be loaded from the network in combination with the programs to display or manipulate them.

Central Processing Unit Operations

The central processing unit sequentially executes program instructions that have been placed in central memory. In the first generation of computers, only a single program and a single set of data could be placed in the computer's central memory, a technique called *monoprogramming*. In a *multi-programming* system, a number of programs may be active in central memory (Figure 1.6). Each program represents an execution process, but only one program may be executed at one time. This technique is used in most microcomputers (e.g., Macintosh with the MacOS operating system, IBM PC and compatibles with DOS or Windows). Only one user may work with the computer at a given time.

Processor(s) Programs in memory	One	Several
One	Monoprogramming	
Several	Multiprogramming Time sharing	Multiprocessing Parallel processing

Figure 1.6 : Processing unit operation

In a *time-sharing* system, the CPU successively allocates time slices to each connected user. The system operates so quickly that each user has the impression of being the only one using the system. This technique is used on most mini- and mainframe computers, especially systems using the UNIX or Windows NT operating systems.

The most powerful machines offer *multiprocessing*, where many processors work simultaneously on different programs. Multiprocessing systems currently pose complex problems for synchronizing different tasks and optimizing performance. Currently the number of processors is limited (from two to sixteen). A new generation of computers, built around a "massively parallel" architecture, is currently under development. These systems will use many hundreds or even thousands of processors to handle applications in areas that require large and repetitive calculations (e.g., image processing, voice recognition, text translation, etc.).

Input-Output Peripherals

Entering Text

The most common method for entering text remains the alphanumeric keyboard. Handwriting recognition, optical scanning of documents, and optical character recognition are developing rapidly.

Selecting Objects

Pointing tools such as the mouse, light pen, trackball, or a digitizing pad let the user indicate points or draw outlines, and represent a useful complement to the keyboard. Fingers can also be used on touch screens to indicate menu selections.

Voice Recognition

Human voice recognition should develop rapidly over the next few years. This development is related to the power of computers, which, according to experts, must execute a billion instructions per second in order to enable the recognition of spoken sentences.

Display Screens

The visual display unit is the most common man–machine interface. Graphic screens offer high resolution, ranging from 600×400 up to 2500×2000 points or pixels (*picture elements*). They usually include micro-processors with RAM for storing pixels (*bitmap screens*) and ROM for graphics software.

Voice Output

Voice output offers a useful complement to the visual display or printout of results, especially in work environments where a written record is not necessary.

Printers

Two types of printers dominate the market: dot matrix printers (employing either impact or ink-jet technology) and laser printers, which provide very high print quality. These offer the use of numerous character sets or *fonts*. Each font can be described as a matrix of points (bitmapped fonts) or mathematical figures (outline fonts).

Software Architecture

Different software layers enable the system to manage the interaction between the user and the computer. Figure 1.7 divides this software in three major categories.

Operating Systems

The *Operating System* (OS) is the set of low-level programs that make the computer run (managing central memory and peripherals, executing programs, scheduling tasks, and handling communications between the com-

| **Application programs** |
| Productivity software: word processing, spreadsheets, graphics tools, groupware tools, etc. |
| Specialized programs: medical record management, image processing, computer-based training, etc. |
| **Development environments** |
| Language libraries, interface managers, database management systems, communication tools, etc. |
| **Operating systems** |
| Task management, virtual memory management, peripheral management, etc. |

Figure 1.7 : Major software categories

puter's components and the outside world). Some of the most widely distributed operating systems on mini- and mainframe computers include IBM/VM-CMS, Digital-VMS, UNIX and Windows NT; for microcomputers they include Microsoft DOS/Windows, IBM-OS2, Mac OS, and Linux. The operating system maintains the directory of files that are stored in memory (i.e., programs and data). Some operating systems provide virtual memory management, which can split working memory for a process between fast central memory and slower peripheral memory.

Development Environments and Utilities

Utilities and development tools are designed for programmers responsible for developing applications. These tools include compilers and interpreters for programming languages, interface management systems, database management systems, and various communication tools. The principles of software development and the tools used are described in detail in the next chapter.

Programming Languages

The computer's central processor executes instructions encoded in *machine language,* or binary language, and stored in the computer's memory. Each computer processor is able to execute a limited number of binary instructions (e.g., addition, subtraction, complements) that are specific to the given processor. RISC-based computers (reduced instruction set computer), which make up the new generation of systems, use a very limited set of elementary instructions that may be executed at very high speeds, in contrast with the previous generation called CISC (complex instruction set computer).

The difficulty of programming in binary language led programmers to develop several generations of *artificial languages* for programming, characterized by a precisely defined syntax and semantics, with a high level of abstraction:

- *Assembly languages*, developed at the same time as the first computers, let programmers use alphabetical operation codes and represent operands in the form of symbols. They are specific to a given processor.
- Third-generation languages (3GL) were developed during the 1960s. They use natural-language words and a processor-independent syntax. The program instructions in a third-generation language are transformed into a machine-executable language. This translation can be carried out either for the entire program, using a *compiler* that transforms the original instructions into an executable object, or on a step-by-step basis by an *interpreter* that can execute the instructions as they are translated. COBOL, C, C++, FORTRAN, and Pascal are examples of compiled languages. BASIC, Java, LISP, MUMPS, and SmallTalk are interpreted. A program written with a 3GL may be compiled or interpreted on computers made by different manufacturers (portability).
- *Fourth-generation languages* (4GL) are higher-level languages designed to facilitate data management and generate reports. They are usually associated with database management systems (DBMS) (see Chapter 2).

Interface Management

The man–machine interface largely determines the success of an information system. In theory, an interface must be natural, efficient, reliable, and easy to understand and to use; in other words, as close as possible to the various human methods of perception and communication such as speech and writing. The Macintosh presented a significant advance in this area. It helped to define a set of conventions for presentation and actions (e.g., how to select, open, or save a file).

Interfaces manage three types of interaction that may be combined: command languages, menu systems, and the direct manipulation of objects.

- A *command language* typically takes the form of a verb followed by the name of an object and optional qualifiers or arguments of the verb. Many computer operating systems and database management systems use command languages. For example, the `dir *.doc` command of the DOS operating system displays the list of files whose names end with `.doc`.
- *Menu systems* present the possible choices on the screen, eliminating or reducing the learning phase.
- *Direct manipulation* was made popular by the Apple Macintosh desk metaphor (Figure 1.8). Interaction takes place using the mouse. The user carries out operations on one or several objects that may be represented as text, graphics, or symbols (e.g., an icon).

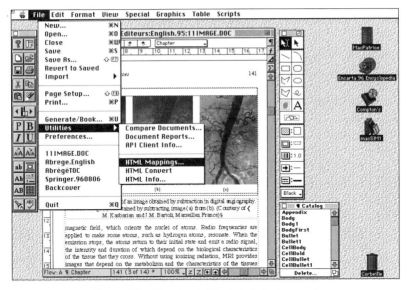

Figure 1.8 : The Apple Macintosh desk metaphor

Application Programs

Application programs are designed for users who are not programmers. Productivity software (e.g., word processing, spreadsheets, drawing tools, or presentation tools), groupware tools (e.g., electronic mail or E-mail), and statistical software are not specific to a given domain. The principal application areas in medicine, such as management of medical records, decision support systems, or computer-based training, are illustrated in Figure 1.9. They are discussed further in later chapters.

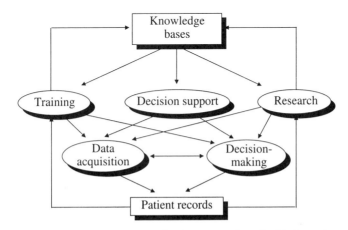

Figure 1.9 : The principal application areas of medical informatics

Communications and Networks

Network Architecture

The development of telecommunications has progressively enabled the creation of computer networks. Connections can be made through electrical cabling, optical fibers, or over the Hertzian waves. Each resource connected to the network is available to all the users who are connected to that network. This access requires knowledge of the location of each application on computers in a *decentralized system*, or may become transparent on a *distributed system*.

Two types of networks may be distinguished by the topology of their connections:

- Computers in a *point-to-point network* are linked together two-by-two to create a star, lattice, or hierarchical structure (Figure 1.10). When low throughputs are sufficient (a few kilobytes per second) a point-to-point link between two remote computers may use modems and the telephone network.

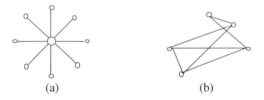

$$(a) \qquad\qquad\qquad (b)$$

Figure 1.10 : Point-to-point networks, (a) star, (b) lattice

- In *broadcast networks*, messages emitted by one computer are sent to all computers in the network. The network topology may be a bus (e.g., Ethernet allows a rate of 10 Mbits and, more recently, 100 Mbits and 1 Gbits per second); a token ring (e.g., IBM Token Ring at 16 Mbits per second); or may use a communication system based on radio waves or satellite distribution. Several local area networks and wide-area networks use this type of architecture (Figure 1.11).

Two types of networks may be distinguished according to the area covered by the network:

- *Local area networks* (LAN) link several computing resources located from a few meters to a few kilometers apart, with transmission speeds ranging from a few megabits to several gigabits per second.
- *Wide area networks* (WAN) link resources or sets of resources located from a few kilometers to tens of thousands of kilometers apart for satellite transmissions. The ARPANET network, created in 1969 on an initiative of the U.S. Department of Defense Research Projects Agency

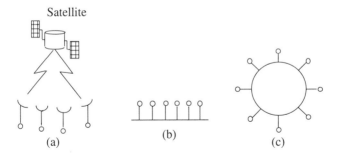

Figure 1.11 : Multipoint or broadcast networks
(a) Satellite distribution, (b) bus structure, (c) ring structure

(DARPA) is one of the very first long-distance networks that let researchers and government employees exchange messages or data files. Transmission speeds on a wide area network range from tens of thousands of kilobits per second to a few million bits per second. The development of high-speed, long-distance connections have enabled the creation of the *information superhighway.*

Today, the interconnection of local area networks by high-speed communication lines has enabled the development of *cyberspace* and allows millions of individuals around the planet to exchange multimedia information.

Standards for Exchanging Information

Establishing Standards

The ability to connect computers from various origins, combined with user demand for portable applications on heterogeneous machines, led to the development of communication *protocols,* or rules, for connection and communication. In some cases, the standards adopted were imposed by the market. These are called *de facto* standards. In other cases, international standards organizations have created *de jure* standards based on recommendations from groups of experts. The increased hardware and software compatibility provided by standards encourages market growth and improved competition [De Moor 1993].

The International Standard Organization (ISO) is the principal worldwide organization for standards. It has proposed a networking standard based on a seven-layer model, from the physical layer to the application layer. This model is called the OSI model (*Open systems interconnection*).

The Consultative Committee on International Telegraphy and Telephony (CCITT) is an international organization responsible for studying and developing recommendations concerning telecommunications (e.g., protocols for data transmission, error correction, or data compression).

In the United States, the American National Standards Institute (ANSI), the American Society for Testing Materials (ASTM) and the Institute of Electrical and Electronics Engineers (IEEE) are particularly active in this area [Hammond 1995].

In Europe, standardization efforts are federated by the *Comité Européen de Normalisation* (CEN) and in particular by the Technical Committee 251 (CEN/TC251) for the health sector [De Moor 1995].

Communication Protocols

TCP/IP (Transmission Control Protocol/Internet Protocol), developed by DARPA in the 1970s, is the most widely used protocol on the Internet. Data to be transmitted between two computers are divided into packets of a few hundred characters. Control information and the addresses of the transmitting and receiving computers are added to the packets. They may be routed in any order, but must be reordered upon arrival. The public nature of the TCP/IP protocol and its availability on multiple hardware platforms (from hand-held computers to mainframes) explain its success.

The X.25 protocol from the CCITT is another example of a packet transmission protocol, based on the concept of connection. Before transmitting data, a virtual transmission circuit is established depending on the availability of the transmitting computers (routers). This method was used for the ATM (asynchronous transfer mode) protocol, the basis for several projects for the information superhighway. The debits supported by ATM (a few Mbits per second to a few hundred Mbits per second) enable the simultaneous transmission of data, voice, and audio-video signals.

The X.400 protocol from the CCITT defines the basis for transporting messages in which the message contents are associated with a message header and inserted in an envelope designed for the transport system. The system generates a receipt when the message has arrived.

Integrated System Architectures

Centralized Systems

These various hardware, software, and communication possibilities let specialists design different architectures to allocate resources and services between computer systems. Figure 1.12 illustrates a centralized architecture. The central computer supplies all the services: communications between workstations, data storage, calculations, etc. This model requires that all software runs on the same computer.

Centralized systems group all useful information on a single computer and facilitate the installation of backup and access procedures to guarantee the security of the information system. The major disadvantage is the archi-

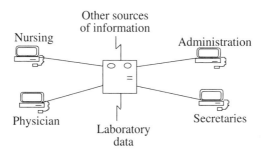

Figure 1.12 : Centralized architecture

tecture's lack of flexibility, which does not allow simple evolution and makes the institution dependent on a single computer manufacturer.

Distributed Systems

Figure 1.13 presents a distributed architecture using specialized local servers to store certain types of information (e.g., patient identities, medical data, laboratory results, images) and manage communications or calculations. This approach builds a computing system in successive stages of hardware and/or software components, which may use equipment from different manufacturers. It increases the complexity of the information system, however, and may cause compatibility problems between various hardware and software components as well as security problems. Each computer becomes a potential Trojan horse for entry into the network (e.g., computer virus introduction).

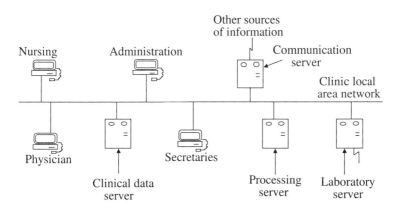

Figure 1.13 : Distributed architecture

Multimedia Workstations

The development of multimedia workstations has become a key element in computer architectures (Figure 1.14). It allows traditional applications to include rich data types (e.g., sound, still images, and animated video sequences) along with the data used in traditional information management. The possibilities for local processing and display facilitate the development of interfaces that hide the complexity of the underlying computer system from the enduser. Finally, access methods such as the smart card may be integrated into the workstation to improve global security for the computing environment.

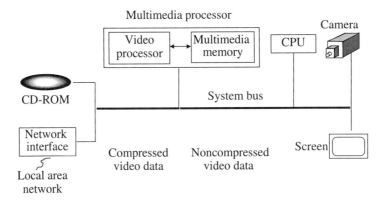

Figure 1.14 : Multimedia architecture (adapted from [Sprague 1992])

The multimedia workstation may progressively fill the role of a camera for image capture, a display or television screen, and a telephone or a videophone, combining these previously disassociated technologies in a single environment [Davis 1991]. The functions of a scanner, printer, copier, and fax may also be grouped together.

Network of Networks

Establishing a network of networks, which ties together the local area networks of the company, changes the concept of the company itself [Tapscott 1993]. Access to the data on the network becomes ubiquitous: at the office via the workstation, at home via personal microcomputers or network computers (teleconsulting and/or teleworking), or via the Hertzian network using a personal assistant equipped with the necessary communications tools. Working in groups (using *groupware*) is enhanced by exchanging messages (e.g., electronic mail or E-mail, group discussions), remote connections, and videoconferencing. Several companies can share resources around a common objective, creating a *virtual company*, as illustrated in Figure 1.15.

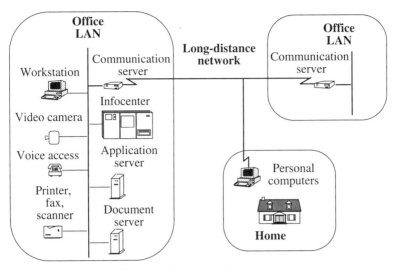

Figure 1.15 : A virtual company

The Internet, initially used by universities and research centers, can virtually connect all world private and public networks. Relying on the TCP/IP protocol, it offers multiple services such as the access to multimedia servers through navigation tools or *browsers*, electronic mail, and distant connection or transfer of data or program files. At the end of 1994, nearly 25,000 networks and 2.5 million computers were connected to the Internet, while traffic increased nearly 10% per month [Laquey 1995]. At the end of 1998, it is estimated that approximately 150 million endusers all over the world are connected. This success and the wide availability and low cost of Internet tools have incited institutions to use the same approach and build local Internet-based networks now called Intranet.

Exercises

- *Explain the differences between informatics and information.*
- *Cite the principal elements of all computers, and describe their respective roles in information processing.*
- *Define the principle of machine coding of information.*
- *Define the concepts of computer programs and programming languages.*
- *Cite the principal software categories.*
- *Discuss some of the difficulties related to managing multimedia information.*

- *Define the concepts of compatibility and standards. Cite a few international standards organizations and examples of standards in the health sector.*
- *Discuss the major computer network architectures and their advantages and disadvantages. Describe some sample networks.*
- *Define the concept of groupware and the virtual enterprise. In this context, what is the role of the workstation?*

2

Medical Software Development

Introduction

The cost of software, both for developing and maintaining programs, represents a growing part of computing budgets and sometimes exceeds hardware costs. The increase in these costs, observed over the past 20 years, is largely due to the growing complexity of the problems to be solved and to the ever-changing requirements of users. Some programs, such as hospital information systems, represent several million lines of code and involve teams of several hundred programmers.

The best way to obtain software that is adapted to one's needs and budget limitations is to perform a detailed initial analysis of the problem to be solved. This helps minimize design errors, reduce development costs, and facilitate future modifications. It is also important to clearly define the methodology for developing a complex computer program and to select techniques that will improve the productivity of the development teams.

A methodology is a kind of guide, a manual for an application development project. A technique is a particular method for carrying out specific tasks. The first two sections of this chapter are devoted to methodology, while the last two deal with technical tools and their integration.

Computer Project Management

Waterfall Models

Most methods used for managing computer projects divide development into phases or steps separated by control points. A step may not be started until the previous step has been validated at a control point. The *waterfall model*, which dates back to the early 1960s, is the best known. Figure 2.1 illustrates the phases in the model:

1. *Requirement analysis* defines the objectives of the computer system and specifies user requirements. The problem is defined: the WHY of the computer system.

2. The *specification* phase defines user requirements in terms of the functionality of the computing system as seen from the outside: the WHAT of the system.

3. The *design* phase provides a precise model of the system and a detailed description of its implementation. It defines the HOW of the system. It is often divided into two steps, the architectural design step and the detailed design step leading to a formalism that will enable program coding.

4. The *implementation* or *development* phase concerns the writing of the program code.

5. The *validation* phase concerns the installation and testing of the system in a real usage situation.

6. *Maintenance* concerns the updating and successive improvements that must be performed on the system.

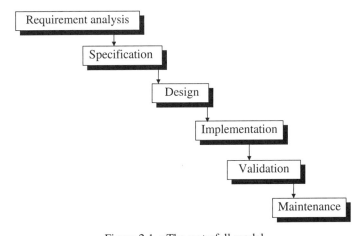

Figure 2.1 : The waterfall model

The MERISE method, widely used in France for the design of information systems, is based on the waterfall method [Nanci 1992]. It defines the following six phases:

1. The first phase concerns the *strategic plan* which identifies and specifies the perspectives of future operations of the enterprise, sets the development priorities, and determines the corresponding schedule and budget.

2. The second phase covers the *preliminary design*. This phase defines the architecture for the functional and technical solutions. It produces the general functional specifications.

3. The *detailed design* phase describes the functional specifications in exhaustive detail. It produces the detailed functional specifications of the application and defines the techniques to be used.

4. The *development* phase starts with a technical study of the programs and organizes them in modules. It continues with the writing of the programs and the corresponding tests.

5. The *implementation* phase covers the various accompanying measures. It is concluded with the *reception* of the application.

6. The *follow-up* (or *maintenance*) process verifies that the services rendered correspond to the services required and guarantees the evolution of the product. It may lead to a new detailed study or to updates to the master plan.

The RACINES (the acronym for *RAtionalisation des Choix INformatiquEs*) guide published by the French Industry Ministry formalizes the definition and implementation of the strategic plan [MRI 1988]. It proposes the following five steps:

1. The first step is the *opportunity and preparation study* of the strategic plan. It includes the implementation of the working organization, usually organized around a *management committee,* which acts as the decision-making body, a *user group* or consulting body, and a *project group,* which plays the role of the general contractor or producer.

2. The *appraisal and orientation* step analyzes the information systems and existing resources; defines the needs, the stakes and the priorities; and determines the direction to be taken.

3. The next step concerns the *scenarios.* A scenario is a strategy that fulfills the objectives set by the strategic plan. Each scenario that is developed includes a conceptual solution, an organization solution, a technical solution, a financial evaluation, sequencing that reflects priorities, and an evaluation of the main impact of the scenario on the organization. Only one scenario is chosen.

4. The objective of step 4, the *action plan*, is to develop a progressively detailed and quantified description of the scenario chosen in step 3. For each action plan, the consequences for the organization and the operation of the services in question are evaluated, along with the technical and human resources required.

5. The last step is the *implementation* and *follow-up* of the strategic plan.

Most master plans require 6 to 18 months, while action plans span a period from 5 to 10 years.

Waterfall methods correspond rather well to the intuitive vision of the development of a computerized system. It is important to specify a system first in general terms, then in more detail, before starting development. The control points, executed between each step, validate the work that has been accomplished. There are several disadvantages, however:

- The method does not always account for the necessary resources or the quality control processes for the products supplied at each step.
- The method is poorly suited to large projects where specifications may change.

Software engineering techniques, discussed later, have progressed considerably. They now rapidly provide significant results in the form of prototypes that may be presented directly to users.

Spiral Methods and Quick Prototyping

Spiral methods are based on the principle of incremental development. New functions are added at each increment. Each loop in the spiral includes requirement analysis, specification, design, implementation, and validation phases (Figure 2.2). At the end of each loop, a new version of the software is produced, which will be supported by specific maintenance.

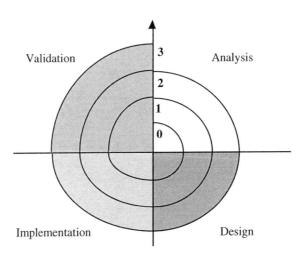

Figure 2.2 : The spiral model

Spiral methods and quick prototyping help improve management of the resources assigned to a project. They emphasize the development of a version of a system, and allow a precise validation and verification of each developed version. Cascading errors (initial design errors that are propagated during future development stages) are always possible, but the method makes it relatively simple to return to the last acceptable version of the program.

Conceptual Models

The Notion of a Model

The notion of a *model* appears in nearly all phases of software development. A model is an idealized vision of reality, an *abstraction* that masks certain details to bring forth others. We can define mathematical models, physical models, and biological models, to name a few. A computer model is a model designed to facilitate the process of developing information systems and software.

To define the *structural properties* of a model is to describe its "anatomy", how the model is organized, what it is made from. An organism is made up of organs, an organ of cells, etc. But be careful: a model only makes sense at a given level of analysis. If we greatly increase the magnification, the concept of a cell becomes much less clear. The separation between a cell and its neighbor is not so clear. At other levels of magnification, we find sets of molecules, atoms, particles, and so on.

To define the *behavioral properties* of a model is to define its "physiology", what it does or how it reacts in response to external stimuli.

Computer models are concerned with the structural and behavioral properties of data, information, and knowledge.

Normally, *data* are the elementary facts that are recorded concerning the phenomena of the outside world and may be considered as given. A patient's temperature of 37.5 ° C is a data item.

Information may be defined as the increase in knowledge that may be deduced from a set of data, from the raw material that facts represent.

Knowledge is the result of successive additions of information to the initial data, information that itself is considered as data for the inferences of higher levels. The distinction between data, information and knowledge is obviously relative.

When we mention interpretation, we refer to the interpreter, that is, the person (the physician, the nurse) or the machine that, based on data, deduces new information and knowledge. Computer-based modeling must take account of the actors in the process and the methods of reasoning used (see Chapter 4).

Having defined these concepts, the major components of computer-based modeling can be defined as follows:

- identify the environment (the WHERE), the players involved in the model (the WHO), and the reasons for the model (the WHY);
- identify the objects of the model, their granularity (the smallest element considered), and their structural and comportmental properties (the HOW);
- validate the model and adapt it so that it better represents the problem at hand.

Objects and Relationships

An *object* is a component of a computer-based model. An object may, (in the case of concrete object) or may not (in the case of abstract object) exist physically. Consider the following example summary of a patient record.

> M. Jones, 43 years old, was hospitalized at Broussais Hospital on June 16, 1998, for a coronary thrombosis. A heparin treatment was prescribed upon admission.

Mr. Jones and the Broussais Hospital may be considered as concrete objects, while the concepts of a patient, a hospital, a diagnosis, and a treatment are abstract objects. In general, the nouns in a sentence describing a given situation are likely candidates for creating the object categories of a model.

Defining objects is not enough, however. We must also define the relationships between objects. The principal role of the verbal groups is to describe these relationships. The preceding example indicated that Mr. Jones *is–treated* with heparin and inversely that heparin *treats* Mr. Jones, that Mr. Jones *is–aged* 43 years and that 43 years *is–the–age–of* Mr. Jones.

Based on these observations, two major approaches for modeling may be defined. The first approach, which favors the objects (the names) and attempts to build elementary structures, may be called the database approach. The second favors the relationships between objects (the verbs). It is mainly used in artificial intelligence as a basis for creating semantic networks and conceptual graphs.

Modeling Intermediate Structures

In the database approach, certain categories of objects may be considered as properties of other objects, which will be emphasized. In the preceding example, age may be defined as a property of the patient object.

An *elementary data item*, the smallest quantity of information that can be manipulated, may be represented as a quadruplet:

<object name, object property, property value, time>

Thus, for the preceding example, we obtain:

<Mr. Jones, age, 43 years, 16 June 1998>.

This representation assumes that time is clearly defined, which is not always the case. For example, we may know that event *A* preceded event *B* without knowing the exact date at which each event occurred.

The grouping or aggregation of the various properties of an object, which are called the *attributes* of the object, allows construction of *elementary data structures*. The relationship linking the object and its property has been rendered implicit: it is now part of the elementary structure. Elementary structures may be linked together to form more complex structures, which may in turn be linked together, much as Lego blocks are joined together to form larger structures.

Simple object	Complex object
- integer (e.g., number of children) - real (e.g., body weight) - exclusive list (e.g., yes/no) - character (e.g., "A") - pixel	- image (2D, 3D, animation) - graphics - sound - physiological signal
Compound object	Composite object
- date - character string (e .g., "Dallas") - nonexclusive list (e.g., headaches, sweating, palpitations) - vector (e.g., induced hyperglycemia) - table - aggregate	- aggregate - record - file

Figure 2.3 : Nature and types of various object categories.

Figure 2.3 illustrates this process of building complex objects from more primitive ones. For example, a data item may consist of a set of three integers. A vector is a set of integers or reals (e.g., the different glycemic values collected during an induced hyperglycemia examination). An *aggregate* is a set of elements or items that may be of a different nature (e.g., integers, reals, dates). A *record* is a set of aggregates, some of which may be repeated (e.g., a patient's various visits (see Figure 2.4).

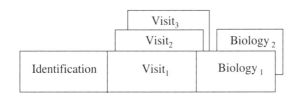

Figure 2.4 : Structure of a record containing two repetitive aggregates (Visit and Biology)

Semantic Networks

Certain verbs or verbal groups are particularly useful for modeling. The verbal groups *is–a* and *is–a–kind–of* may be used to assign an object to a category or class of objects, or to indicate that a class is part of a more general class. Thus Mr. Jones *is-an* instance of the PATIENT object class. A PATIENT *is–a–kind–of* PERSON, a subset of the class PERSON. By successive *generalizations* we can build hierarchies or networks of classes. The objects of a class inherit the properties of the more general class. A person has a name and therefore a patient, a subset of the class person, has a name. The inverse of generalization is called *specialization*.

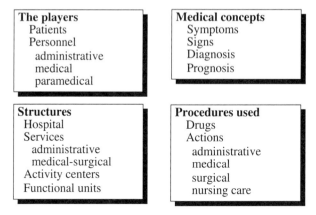

The players
  Patients
  Personnel
    administrative
    medical
    paramedical

Medical concepts
  Symptoms
  Signs
  Diagnosis
  Prognosis

Structures
  Hospital
  Services
    administrative
    medical-surgical
  Activity centers
  Functional units

Procedures used
  Drugs
  Actions
    administrative
    medical
    surgical
    nursing care

Figure 2.5 : Some categories of medical concepts

The verbal group *is–part–of* lets us model the constitution of an object from its constituents. The left ventricle *is–part–of* the heart. Figure 2.5 provides a few examples of *categories* of medical objects, and Figure 2.6 shows examples of relationships between objects.

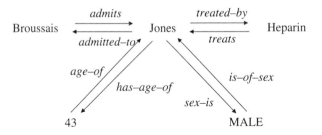

Figure 2.6 : Networked structure

Software Development Tools

Computer-Aided Software Engineering

Software engineering is the set of computer programming techniques that automates the various phases in software development. A *software engineering environment* (SEE) may be defined as a computer system that provides support for the development, debugging, and improvement of software programs, and for the management and control of these activities. The goal is to assist applications developers in all the phases of the development cycle(s) and to improve the productivity of development teams.

SEE assembles the various tools required for software production, including:

- the specification, analysis, and design of target applications;
- the identification and selection of software components (parts of programs) that have already been developed;
- the adaptation and specialization of reusable components or the development of new components;
- the management of the documentation associated with the development in order to facilitate future maintenance and reutilization;
- the definition and management of hardware and software configurations that will execute the applications;
- the validation and evaluation of the components developed.

Rapid prototyping, made possible by SEE tools, enables the realization or the modeling of parts of the system to be developed, which may then be quickly shown to potential users. Figure 2.7 illustrates the interaction that can be achieved between users and application developers. Users' suggestions are integrated in the successive versions of the software.

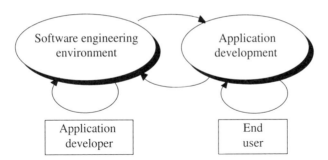

Figure 2.7 : The retroactive loops in software development

Database Management Systems

Definitions

A *database* may be defined as a structured, nonredundant collection of data and the relationships that associate that data, stored on computer-readable media and designed to serve several applications. A database is created to record facts or events concerning individuals or objects, to provide that data upon request, and to create new knowledge based on accumulated data (inferences).

An *intelligent database* may be defined as a database enriched with certain properties of human intelligence, that is:

- it has an intelligent user interface that lets the user communicate with the computer using a quasi-natural language;
- it allows users to access pertinent information by specifying that information without making reference to its physical location on magnetic media;
- it is able to infer knowledge about recorded facts or to compare new situations with the memory of recorded facts.

A *database management system* (DBMS) is a set of programs that allows the user to interact with the database [Date 1995]. A DBMS represents a sort of window between the users and the file management system of the host computer that handles data stored in secondary memory (Figure 2.8).

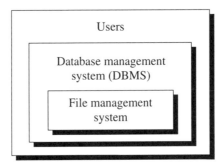

Figure 2.8 : Database management system

General Architecture

Databases are usually defined on three levels:

- The *conceptual level* describes a global model of reality. It is defined by the integration of the partial views of each user or user group (Figure 2.9). The conceptual level describes the different entities managed by the model (e.g., hospitals, hospital services, patients, and staff) and the relationships or associations between those entities. The description of the conceptual model includes a description of the authorized structures (objects and relations between objects) as well as a description of the constraints imposed upon those structures.
- The *external level* is a subset of the general model, called the *view* of each user or set of users. There are potentially an infinite number of views for a given general model.
- The *internal level* corresponds to the structures used to store the information, that is, how the data is stored on the peripheral devices.

Models Used by DBMS

The oldest DBMS are based on the *hierarchical model* and the *network model*.

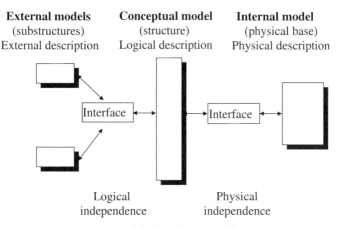

Figure 2.9 : Database model

A *hierarchical* or tree structure is built from an initial element called the root and elements that depend on the root, called the branches. Each branch may in turn be subdivided into subbranches, and so on. The terminal elements are called leaves. Each subdivision represents a level. The root is often considered as level 0. A given node of any level n can have only one parent on level $n-1$. As illustrated in Figure 2.10, the hierarchical model lends

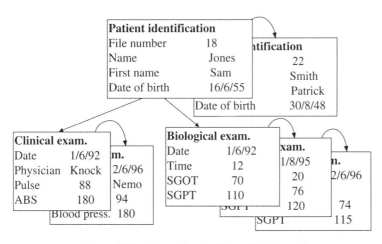

Figure 2.10 : Example of a hierarchical model

itself rather well to a data organization centered around the patient (the root of the tree). It can optimize certain types of access, and in particular order, temporal information such as different visits by the same patient.

Network structures are those where each node of the network may have several parents.

The *relational model*, developed by Codd in the 1970s, owes its success to its extreme simplicity and to the existence of a standardized description and Structured Query Language (SQL) [Codd 1990]. The relational model was the basis of a large number of commercial relational database management systems (RDBMS). A relational model takes the form of a table called a *relation*. Each line in a relation, or *tuple*, has a unique identification key. No tuple may be redundant in a relation. Figure 2.11 illustrates this model using the same example as in Figure 2.10. Unfortunately, RDBMSs are not

Identification

File #	Name	First	Birthdate
18	Jones	Sam	16/6/55
22	Smith	Patrick	30/8/48

Biological examination

File #	Date	Time	SGOT	SGPT
18	1/6/92	12	70	110
18	1/8/95	20	76	120
18	2/6/96	10	74	115

Physician

Name	First	Address
Knock	Gaston	Paris
Nemo	Jules	Argiusta

Clinical examination

File #	Date	Physic.	Pulse	BP
18	1/6/92	Knock	88	180
18	2/6/96	Nemo	94	180

Figure 2.11 : Example of a relational model

well suited to managing temporal data, representing the knowledge associated with the data, managing complex objects such as text or images, or modeling actions or procedures.

Semantic models and models built around the concept of the *frame* [Minsky 1975] attempt to make relations between the elements of the world explicit, that is, to include these relationships in the model's structure. They may be used as a basis for medical knowledge and more elaborate models of medical records.

Object-oriented models are a good compromise between purely semantic models and record-based models (i.e., hierarchical, network, and relational models) [Cattel 1994]. Simple or complex objects, such as free text or images, are organized in classes and subclasses. Each class inherits the properties of its parent classes (*simple inheritance*) or of several classes (*multiple inheritance*). Objects exchange *messages*. A model is created for an application by specializing pre-existing object classes and/or by building from primitive objects. A standardized description and query language called OQL has been proposed by the *Object Management Group* (OMG). Object-oriented models and database management systems (ODBMS) are well suited for representing and managing multimedia data.

Document Management Systems

Document management covers not only text, graphics, and images but also sounds or video sequences and, in general, complex objects grouped under the category multimedia. The linear structure of printed documents, which has characterized our civilization for thousands of years, is poorly suited to providing easy access to these various types of information. The concept of *hypertext* has overthrown this traditional view of the written word by offering the possibility of multiple access within and navigation through a document. Hypertext may be considered as a set of nodes (cards in the HyperCard system on the Apple Macintosh) connected via links. The user can access different nodes using an index and may move around the network following multiple paths. Specialized languages, such as the HyperCard language, may be used to describe the conditions for the passage and/or the execution of procedures if certain conditions have been met.

Hypermedia is a hypertext with nodes that may contain multimedia objects such as images or sounds. The approach is particularly useful for creating complex documents (e.g., technical documents) or interactive encyclopedias. Creating multimedia documents and accessing and transmitting them requires the definition of modes for representation, of navigation tools, and of transfer protocols.

Hypermedia document servers in the Internet environment, which may include text, images, sound, and video, use the HTML (*HyperText Markup Language)* to describe documents and the links between them. The Java interpreted language allows the writing of interactive pieces of code, or *applets,* that bring interactivity and dynamicity to HTML pages. The *virtual reality modeling language* (VRML) is a complementary language to represent and manipulate three-dimensional objects. The XML (*Extensible Markup Language*), a subset of the SGML (*Standard Generalized Markup Language*) has been recently proposed formal language that can be used to pass information about the component parts of a document to another computer system. XML is flexible enough to be able to describe any logical text structure, whether it be a form, memo, letter, report, book, encyclopedia, dictionary or database.

Document servers connected via hypertext links in the Internet network make up the *World-Wide Web* (WWW), or simply the Web, a hypermedia library distributed across the planet. Links are established by indicating the document's symbolic address or URL (*Uniform Resource Locator*). A set of useful URL addresses related to medicine is provided in Appendix C. The transfer protocol for Web documents is called the HTTP *(HyperText Transfer Protocol)*. Navigation tools, known as *Internet browsers,* such as Netscape® or Microsoft Internet Explorer®, allow the display of the different Web pages and, if necessary, the execution of the associated applets.

Interface Management Systems

The user interface represents a crucial element in the use of any computer system and to a large extent determines its success. Developing well-adapted interfaces becomes extremely complex and takes up an ever-increasing part of application development. Some studies show that more than 75% of all application code deals with the interface.

Ideally, an interface should be intuitive, easy-to-use, and accessible to nonspecialists. It must clearly present the necessary and available information in the most appropriate form, reflect the status of work in progress, highlight important results, and present warnings. The interface must be adapted to medical users' work methods, which feature frequent interruptions. It is therefore important to be able to interrupt an action, save the state of the interface at the time of the interruption, then easily return to the configuration later.

From a technical viewpoint, the interface must visually represent the different types of medical objects (text, graphics, and images) and eventually include audio and video extensions (i.e., voice control, audio capture or the production of audio documents, and synchronization of sound and images).

The various programs available to the user must share the same environment and look and feel. This homogeneous presentation reduces the time required to learn how to use the application. This has led developers to adopt rules for presentation and style, such as those proposed by the X Windows/Motif standard. The most recent generation of user interface management systems offer multiwindowing, direct object manipulation, and access to multimedia documents.

Natural Language Processing Tools

The advantage of functions for processing medical language is twofold. In a well defined (medical) domain, the automatic analysis of natural language text (e.g., the letter of the practitioner or a report of a procedure) can extract symbolic representations (in the form of graphs, for example), which may be queried at a later date [Baud 1992]. The same representative models may be used to query documentary databases or knowledge bases, making them more accessible to nonspecialists [Rassinoux 1998].

Specialized Software Components

Other components are specific to a particular area of use, or even certain categories of personnel such as intensive care physicians or radiologists. These may be statistical tools, physiological signal processing, images, or decision-support modules that may be integrated in medical applications.

Electronic Data Interchange

Communication functions provide access to all types of medical information at various locations. They enable access to data servers and/or intra- or inter-hospital servers, as well as communication (charts or messaging) between personnel in the health-care system who may be located inside or outside the hospital.

Electronic data interchange (EDI) is concerned with the contents of messages, not how they are transported through the network. In the United States, as in Europe, different organizations and work groups have attempted to define the various protocols for exchanging hospital data, such as ASTM E1238 for laboratory data, HL7 for hospital information systems or XML for structured documents or messages [Dolin 1998]. The EDIFACT group (*Electronic Data Interchange for Administration Commerce and Transport*), founded in 1987, supplies a global framework for document exchange in different sectors of activity. Its proposals in health care include the standardization of transactions for admission and discharge, requests for and return of complementary examinations, prescriptions for medication, and the transmission of medical data.

Image transmission (e.g., for radiology) presents special problems because of the volume of information to be transmitted and the need to associate clinical data describing the conditions under which the examination took place as well as observations of the results. The American College of Radiology (ACR) in collaboration with the National Electrical Manufacturers Association (NEMA), published a standard for transmitting radiological images, called the ACR/NEMA standard. The latest version, named DICOM, is well suited to sequences of images.

Integrating Software Components

The development of medical software is a complex process that follows a precise methodology using successive additions of software components. This accumulation, however, is not sufficient to create a coherent application. The components must be perfectly integrated. From a technical viewpoint, this integration has at least four aspects:

- *Integration by presentation* guarantees the homogeneity of the presentation and dialogues, and attempts to reduce the user's "cognitive load" by making the passage from one application module to another transparent. It uses presentation standards independent of the operating system and interface building and usage guidelines specific to one or a set of users.
- *Integration by data* concerns sharing information and associated documentation. It is facilitated by the creation of a *metamodel* — a model of all the models used — and a global data dictionary — a description of all the objects used.

- *Integration by communication* concerns the syntax, semantics and pragmatics of messages exchanged between the software components. The goal is to allow interaction between the components without losing information or modifying the meaning. For example, messages sent by the components must be received exactly as sent.
- The objective of *integration by control* is to coordinate the various components (i.e., sequential or parallel processing, automatic triggering of procedures, optimization of strategies, etc.).

Exercises

- *List the principal steps in managing a computer project.*
- *Discuss the pros and cons of the waterfall method and the fast prototyping method.*
- *Explain the principle of a strategic plan.*
- *Define the concepts of data, information and knowledge. Describe the principal elementary data types.*
- *Explain the concepts of model, object, and categories of objects.*
- *List the main software categories required to develop a computer application. What is a SEE system?*
- *What are the main objectives and functions of a database management system? List some models for database management systems.*
- *Define the concepts of hypertext and hypermedia. Cite examples of their use in medicine.*
- *What are the problems involved concerning the exchange of computerized medical data? Cite a few examples of interchange standards for medical data.*
- *Define an integrated medical application.*

3

Medical Data and Semiology

Introduction

Expressions such as "data acquisition" or "gathering information" are employed frequently in the practice of medicine. They may lead one to believe that information is readily available, and it is sufficient to gather it to make a diagnosis and propose a treatment. Indeed, a seemingly objective parameter such as a biological dosage can only be interpreted, in other words become information, by considering the motivation for the prescription, the blood sampling conditions, the method used for measuring, etc. A symptom or a clinical or radiological sign is the result of a complex decision-making process. Health professionals are constantly led to consider one or several hypotheses, then to search for elements that can either confirm or refute them. The hypotheses that are retained will serve as the basis for developing more synthetic information and for making decisions.

Medical information therefore only exists in an interpretative framework that must constantly be updated to avoid diagnostic or therapeutic errors. Semiology is the part of medicine that studies the signs of diseases. The physician's hypothesis guides data collection, and the selection of information judged as "useful" changes with his or her experience. Subjectivity plays a predominant role in medicine. This situation partly explains the nonexhaustive nature of medical records. Information may be missing because the question was never asked (the examination was never carried out) or, on the other hand, the answer may not have been written in the file. A study carried out by Bentsen [Bentsen 1976] showed that up to 40% of the problems identified by observers in a medical setting were not recorded in the record file.

It is therefore important to evaluate the quality of medical data and to be able to appreciate its informational value. This method may be applied to symptoms as well as to clinical, biological, or radiological signs.

The Nature of Medical Data

Medical Data Types

The modeling principles described in Chapter 2 include at least four elements for each medical data item:
- the patient's name (e.g., M. Jones),
- the attribute or the parameter in question (e.g., age),
- the value for that parameter (e.g., 40),
- the time of the observation (e.g., 16 June 1995 at 10:52 A.M.).

The degree of precision for the values of quantitative variables, such as pulse, is determined by the nature of the measurement. The interpretation of these data also depends on the context of the measurement (is the patient lying down or standing?) and the previous state of the patient. A weight loss of 2 kg measured between two visits 15 days apart does not have the same meaning as an identical weight loss during a single renal dialysis session.

It is often necessary to associate several elementary numeric data items to provide a correct interpretation of physiological phenomena. The systolic blood pressure is associated with the diastolic blood pressure; the various values for a hyperglycemic curve form a set of values.

Some variables are *qualitative* and may have two or more values. A response may be exclusive or nonexclusive such as when several responses may be selected from a list. A *binary* or *boolean* qualitative variable is an exclusive variable with two states (e.g., sex may be male or female, the answer to a question may be yes or no).

Several parameters are stored in continuous records. This is the case for physiological signals such as electroencephalograms or electrocardiograms. The data, which may be digitized (see Chapter 10), are associated with an interpretation in free text format. The complex set (text and data) is stored in the computerized medical record. Fixed and moving images are another type of complex data, also associated with comments in free-form text (see Chapter 11).

The free text produced by these various interpretations is built upon a syntax and semantics that can only be understood if it is shared by the various users (i.e., producers and readers). This requirement has led to the creation of nomenclatures and codes to represent medical concepts in an unambiguous fashion (see Chapter 5).

The Variability of Medical Data

The rate at which medical observations can be successfully reproduced depends on the methods used for measurement (*analytic variability*), the observers (*intra-* and *interobserver variability*), and the subject being observed (*intra-* and *interindividual variability*). Relationships between the various types of variability are illustrated in Figure 3.1.

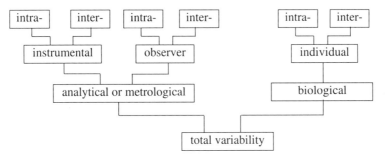

Figure 3.1 : Sources of variability (adapted from [Grémy 1987])

Medical data do not usually provide perfect information and cannot identify diseases with certainty. A data item may stray from the actual value due to imprecision and/or inaccuracy. These two concepts are illustrated in Figure 3.2

- *Precision* refers to the fidelity of the measurement; if the measurement is repeated on the same subject, the same result will be obtained.
- *Accuracy* refers to the tendency of measured values to be symmetrically grouped around the variable's true value.

The fidelity of the measurement of clinical information is difficult to establish, as illustrated in several studies carried out on the analysis of the viewpoints of physicians on identical patient cases.

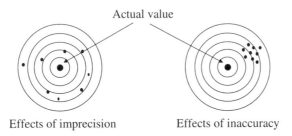

Figure 3.2 : The dispersion of measurements is greater around the central value for imprecision. In the case of inaccuracy, measurements are grouped around a value that is not the one sought.

Interpreting Medical Data

Cognitive Processes

In general, the cognitive process of interpretation uses reasoning by abduction (see Chapter 4), also known as the scientific method. Abduction starts from a suggested hypothesis that explains a given phenomenon and proceeds with successive verifications to confirm or refute the hypothesis. Words used in describing the situations, symptoms, and signs, and the associations established between these signs, have a major influence on this process. This phenomenon, which psychologists call the preconceived notion, is combined with the uncertainty inherent in several diagnostic procedures. It explains in part the *intra-* and *interobserver* variability.

Interpreting Numbers and Words

The absence of a standardized medical vocabulary based on clear definitions makes medical observations fuzzy. The use of close but not strictly synonymous terms for the same concept or for concepts close to the same term is a source of semantic ambiguity and imprecision.

Medical communications, both in medical treatises and in the synthesis of clinical cases, make significant use of qualifiers to quantify certain phenomena. For example, the terms "frequent" or "common" are often used. As Figure 3.3 illustrates, these qualifiers have different meanings to different people.

Qualifiers	Estimated probability	
	Physicians	Non physicians
Associated with	.40	.50
Often	.40	.59
Regularly	.38	.40
Frequently	.50	.45
Occasionally	.30	.33
Typically	.30	.30
Sometimes	.27	.35
Not very often	.25	.28
Seldom	.25	.29
Characteristic	.20	.37
Atypical	.18	.23
Rare	.09	.09

Figure 3.3 : Qualifiers and estimated probabilities (adapted from [Nakao 1983])

Other studies show that the comprehension of numerical terms is also subject to differing interpretations. Numerical estimations do not always result in better communication than qualifiers. These studies illustrate the limits of processing medical information, especially in the form of text. They suggest that precautions should be taken to correctly interpret the results of any study.

Interpreting Associations

The abductive process and diagnostic judgment are based on the frequency of associations between a diagnosis and a particular trait of a description. Several studies show that common events are much more easily perceived than rare ones, and that symptoms and diagnoses may co-occur even if they are not related. These apparent correlations introduce "noise" in the diagnostic reflection process and thereby reduce the quality of the use of data [Schwartz 1986].

Quantitative Semiology

Semiology is the study of signs. *Quantitative semiology* uses tools to evaluate the informational value of medical signs and data.

The Diagnostic Value of a Test

A sign S has a diagnostic value if it can separate sick patients from healthy ones (or disease A from disease B); in other words, if its frequency is significantly different between healthy patients and sick patients (or those who have contracted diseases A and B). The probability P of having disease D if the sign S is present, written $P(D|S)$, is greater than the probability of having D, or the anterior probability of D, written $P(D)$ (Figure 3.4).

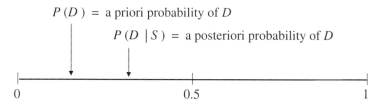

Figure 3.4 : Modification of the probability of a patient being sick by searching for a sign

All medical data do not have the same significance in this diagnostic research. Furthermore, the presence of a sign does not necessarily signify the presence of a disease, and the absence of a sign is not synonymous with the absence of the disease.

The contingency table in Figure 3.5 illustrates the possible situations. We assume there are two populations, one with a given disease D, the other with-

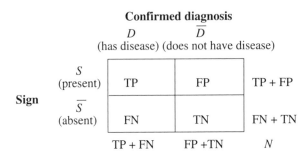

Confirmed diagnosis

	D (has disease)	$\overline{D}$ (does not have disease)	
S (present)	TP	FP	TP + FP
$\overline{S}$ (absent)	FN	TN	FN + TN
	TP + FN	FP +TN	N

Sign

Figure 3.5 : The situations as a function of results from a test. TP = true positive; FP = false positive; TN = true negative; FN = false negative; N = total number of patients.

out, written $\overline{D}$. This certainty has been proven using a reference test called the *gold standard*. The sign S is studied to establish the diagnostic D. Four subgroups may be identified according to the presence (S) or absence ($\overline{S}$) of the sign:

• *true positives* (TP), where both the sign and the disease are present,
• *false positives* (FP), where the sign is present but the disease is absent,
• *false negatives* (FN), who do not present the sign but do have the disease,
• *true negatives* (TN) have neither the sign nor the disease.

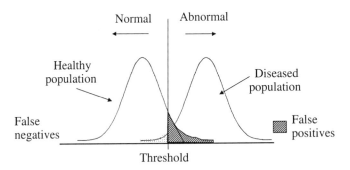

Figure 3.6 : Normality threshold of a test

The same reasoning holds true for known quantitative values if we opt to define a *normality threshold,* labeled Threshold in the example in Figure 3.6. Beyond this threshold the result is considered abnormal. The biological sign is then either present or absent.

The threshold is determined by statistical methods, according to the distribution of the parameter in the population under study. These statistical fluctuations show that the repetition of doses with healthy patients may give abnormal results. The number of abnormal results increases with the number of tests carried out. Figure 3.7 demonstrates that there is a 64% chance for a healthy person to show an abnormal result in an examination including 20 biochemical tests.

Number of tests performed	Probability that at least one test is abnormal (%)
1	5.0
6	26.0
12	46.0
20	64.0
100	99.4

Figure 3.7 : Probability of finding at least one abnormal result for a person in good health (adapted from [Woolf 1990])

The discriminatory value of a biological parameter increases if its distribution is different in both populations under study, as illustrated in Figure 3.8. Test 1 is more discriminating than test 2 because there is less of an overlap between the distributions of the parameter in the healthy population and the diseased population.

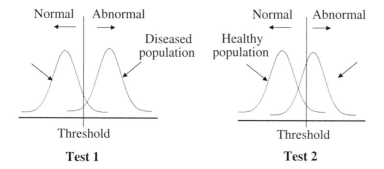

Figure 3.8 : Discriminating ability of two tests. Test 1 is more discriminating than test 2.

Sensitivity and Specificity of a Sign

Sensitivity and specificity are two indicators of the informational value of a medical sign.

Binary Qualitative Sign

For a binary qualitative sign (present or absent), the sensitivity and specificity may be estimated from the contingency table in Figure 3.5. We assume there are two populations, one with a given disease (*D*), the other without ($\overline{D}$).

The *sensitivity (Se)* or *true positive rate* (TPR) is defined as the proportion of patients who show the sign (*S*).

$$Se = \frac{TP}{TP + FN} \tag{3.1}$$

Sensitivity, measured in a sample of patients, is an estimation of the probability of the presence of the sign in those carrying the disease (theoretical sensitivity), written $P(S|D)$.

The *specificity (Sp)* or *true negative rate* (TNR) is defined as the proportion of healthy patients who do not have the sign:

$$Sp = \frac{TN}{(TN + FP)} \tag{3.2}$$

Specificity, measured in a sample of patients who do not have the disease ($\overline{D}$), is an estimation of the probability of the absence of the sign in the healthy population (theoretical specificity), written $P(S|M)$.

A sign is even more specific to a disease *D* if it is rarely observed in patients who do not have the disease. A sign whose specificity is equal to 1 is called *pathognomonic*, such as Köplick's sign for measles.

A good diagnostic test must have high sensitivity and specificity. The following formula represents the *likelihood ratio* (LR):

$$LR = \frac{Se}{(1 - Sp)} \tag{3.3}$$

An ideal sign would have a sensitivity and a specificity of 1. Sensitivity, calculated on a sample of patients who have the disease *D*, and specificity, calculated on a sample of patients who do not have the disease *D*, are independent of the *prevalence* of *D*, which expresses the probability *P(D)* of the disease in the population.

Continuous Quantitative Variables

The evaluation of a biological dosage can be compared to the preceding problem for the choice of a normality threshold. For each value *a* in the selected threshold, we can calculate a value for sensitivity and specificity and find the threshold with the best sensitivity / specificity couple. When the distribution curves of the parameter in the populations *D* and $\overline{D}$ overlap, it is possible to find a threshold offering a sensitivity and a specificity of 1. Any improvement in specificity comes at the expense of sensitivity, and vice versa. The following example illustrates this phenomenon.

The SGOT rate was measured in 94 patients with chest pains. We shall consider the number of cases of coronary thrombosis diagnosed in this sam-

	MI	$\overline{\text{MI}}$			MI	$\overline{\text{MI}}$
SGOT > 100	25	4		SGOT > 120	22	3
SGOT Š 100	23	42		SGOT Š 120	26	43
Total	48	46		Total	48	46

(a) Threshold = 100 Units/l   (b) Threshold = 120 Units/l

Figure 3.9 : Influence of the sensitivity and specificity threshold of SGOT for the diagnosis of myocardial infarction (MI)

ple. Assuming the value of 100 units/l as the threshold above which the test will be considered positive, the sensitivity of the test is 25/48, or 52.1%, and its specificity is 42/46, or 91.3% (Figure 3.9). If we set the threshold at 120 units/l, the sensitivity equals 22/48, or 45.8%, and the specificity is 43/46, or 93.5%.

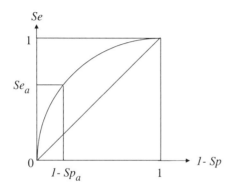

Figure 3.10 : The ROC curve of a test

The informational value of a test compared to a diagnostic may be represented graphically by the curve of $[Se, 1 - Sp]$ pairs, obtained by varying the normality threshold. This curve is called the ROC curve (*receiver-operating characteristic*) (Figure 3.10). Comparing the ROC curves of different tests lets us appreciate the informational value. The test with the best discriminating ability is the one that corresponds to the highest curve (Figure 3.11).

In general, we can say that test *A* is better than test *B* if:

$Se(A) > Se(B)$ and $Sp(A) Š Sp(B)$,

or if

$Sp(A) > Sp(B)$ and $Se(A) Š Se(B)$.

When $Se(A) > Se(B)$ and $Sp(A) < Sp(B)$, it is not possible to classify *A* and *B*.

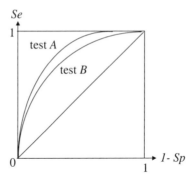

Figure 3.11 : A format for ranking tests. Test *A* is better than test *B*.

Consideration for the Cost of Tests

The method described above does not take into consideration the respective costs of the two possible diagnostic errors: incorrectly ignoring the disease *D* or incorrectly diagnosing *D*. The cost must be considered from two perspectives: the health cost and the financial cost. The *health cost* is measured in terms of mortality or morbidity. The *financial cost* includes the cost of treatment and the costs incurred by the death or the invalidity of the patient.

These costs can only be evaluated in medical, social, and ethical terms. In practice, for a given test, we tend to privilege sensitivity or specificity according to the chosen strategy. We select ill patients or eliminate healthy patients using tests to confirm a diagnosis or to detect a disease.

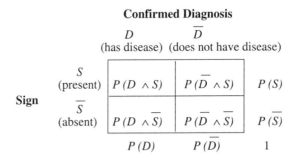

Figure 3.12 : Predictive values of a sign

Measuring the Predictive Value of a Sign

When making a medical decision, it is useful to consider the posterior probability of the disease once the result of the test is known. Following Figure 3.12, we can distinguish four probabilities: $P(D \wedge S)$, $P(D \wedge \bar{S})$, $P(\bar{D} \wedge S)$, and $P(\bar{D} \wedge \bar{S})$.

Knowing that $P(D \wedge S) = P(D) \cdot P(S|D)$, if $P(D)$ is the prevalence of the disease in the general population, we can estimate the positive and negative predictive values of a sign using Bayes' formula (see Appendix A).

The probability $P(D \mid S)$ that an individual who has the sign has contracted the disease is called the *positive predictive value* (PPV) or the *diagnostic value*.

$$\text{PPV} = P(D|S) = \frac{P(D \wedge S)}{P(S)} \tag{3.4}$$

$$\text{PPV} = \frac{P(D) \cdot P(S|D)}{P(D) \cdot P(S|D) + P(\overline{D}) \cdot P(S|\overline{D})} \tag{3.5}$$

However, the probability $P(S|D)$ corresponds to the sensitivity Se and the probability $P(S|D)$ equals $1 - Sp$. Therefore, the estimation of the PPV value may be obtained using the following expression:

$$\text{PPV} = \frac{P(D) \cdot Se}{P(D) \cdot Se + (1 - P(D))(1 - Sp)} \tag{3.6}$$

The probability $P(\overline{D} \mid \overline{S})$ that an individual who does not have the sign also does not have the disease is called the *negative predictive value* (NPV).

$$\text{NPV} = P(\overline{D}|\overline{S}) = \frac{P(D \wedge S)}{P(\overline{S})} \tag{3.7}$$

$$\text{NPV} = \frac{P(\overline{D}) \cdot P(\overline{S}|\overline{D})}{P(\overline{D}) \cdot P(\overline{S}|\overline{D}) + P(D) \cdot P(\overline{S}|D)} \tag{3.8}$$

Hence we can conclude:

$$\text{NPV} = \frac{(1 - P(D)) \cdot Sp}{(1 - P(D)) \cdot Sp + P(D) \cdot (1 - Se)} \tag{3.9}$$

The diagnostic value is equal to:
- 1 if $Sp = 1$, that is, if the sign is pathognomonic;
- $P(D)$ if $S_e = 1 - S_p$, that is, if the sign has no diagnostic value for disease D (if the probability of having the disease does not change with the presence or the absence of the sign).

If A is better than B (i.e., $S_e(A) > S_e(B)$ and $S_p(A) > S_p(B)$), then the diagnostic value of A is greater than that of B.

The positive predictive value lets us evaluate a sign in a positive diagnostic situation because it only accounts for one type of error: false positives. If we consider the two predictive values at the same time, then sign A is preferable to sign B if PVP(A) > PVP(B) and, simultaneously, PVN(A) > PVN(B). In practice, the two situations rarely occur simultaneously.

Equations (3.4) to (3.9) show that evaluating the predictive values of a sign for a disease D depends on the prevalence of disease D. The prevalence is often difficult to determine in diagnostic situations where the patient cannot be considered as having been selected at random from the general population. It may be difficult to estimate the a priori probability that the patient carries the disease.

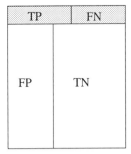

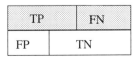

Sample (frequency of the
disease = 0.5)

Total population (frequency
of the disease << 0.5)

Figure 3.13 : Effect of prevalence in the population and the sample studied
(adapted from [Weinstein 1980])

Figure 3.13, taken from Weinstein [Weinstein 1980], illustrates the relationship between the distribution of test results in the total population and in the observed sample.

As demonstrated in Figure 3.14, if the prevalence is less than 1%, the positive predictive value of a test is low despite good sensitivity and good specificity.

Discussion and Conclusions

The indicators and the informational value of a sign are extremely useful for developing a diagnostic strategy. In any case, evaluation studies of these indicators are often biased. They can only be used after having answered the following questions [Philbrick 1980]:

1. Has the population description been studied to the point where the results may be used in my practice?
2. Are the subjects examined in the sample studied comparable to the patients whom I wish to test?
3. What is the value of the gold standard for the chosen test? Does it let me establish the state of the patient with certainty?
4. Was the interpretation of the gold standard carried out blindly?
5. Were the analyzed data obtained by several independent observers? If

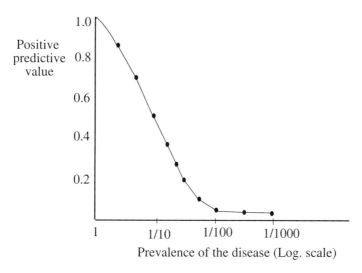

Figure 3.14 : Relation between the prevalence and the positive predictive value
(sensitivity and specificity at 90%)

so, how was the problem of disagreements between the various observers handled?

The validity of the indicators depends on the methodology and the rigor
used when the data were gathered. As when evaluating any problem, the goal
must be clearly stated. This lets us define the diseases studied, the conditions
for testing, and applicability and interpretation of the test being evaluated.
Bias must be systematically identified and avoided. Prevalence effects must
be carefully studied.

Exercises

- *What are the major types of medical data?*
- *Define and characterize the variable nature of medical data.*
- *Evaluate the diagnostic or predictive value of a test or a sign.*
- *Define true positive, true negative, false positive, and false negative
  rates.*
- *Define the concepts of sensitivity, specificity, and likelihood ratio.*
- *Define a ROC curve.*
- *Compare the informational value of two tests.*
- *Critically analyze the results of a study on the informational value of a
  test.*

4

Medical Reasoning and Decision-Making

Introduction

Decision-making is the physician's essential activity. In theory, making a decision involves creating a list of possible strategies and/or actions, determining the consequences of each decision, and selecting the most appropriate solution for the context. But things rarely happen this way in medicine. Basic medical information is often imperfect, subjective, or unspecific. There are too many possible hypotheses to consider each one individually. Only fragmentary knowledge of the consequences of each decision is available, and the foreseeable effects of treatment can only be guessed at. Medical decisions are made under uncertainty. They present a judgment that is generally a preference for a solution or a treatment that has been deemed optimal. The objective of the medical process is to reduce uncertainty by acquiring complementary information through the use of diverse and complex knowledge.

Computers may assist in medical decision-making and improve the quality of diagnosis or the efficiency of therapy. Creating systems to assist in medical decision-making requires considerable thought in order to formalize the problem and the possible solutions. This research helps us better understand the mechanisms involved in medical reasoning and the elaboration of the knowledge that supports that reasoning. This chapter presents an overview of the principles of medical reasoning, an analysis of the characteristics of medical decisions, and, finally, different computer-based methods for representing knowledge and decision support systems.

Reasoning

Deduction

Deductive reasoning is based on the principles of logical implication. It allows us to infer conclusions, the degree of truth of which is only a function of the degree of truth of the premises. Deduction works from the general to the specific. If the rule "all men are mortal" is true, then Socrates, who is a man, is mortal (*modus ponens*). The results of logical inference may be used as a premise for further deductions. Thus, if *A* implies *B* and if *B* implies *C*, then, via transitivity, *A* implies *C*.

Deductive reasoning is based on logical rules or absolute knowledge that lets us relate propositions (Figure 4.1). A review of propositions and predicate logic is provided in Appendix B. In these types of logic, propositions are either *true* or *false*.

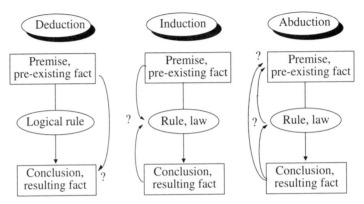

Figure 4.1 : Different types of reasoning

Induction

Inductive reasoning makes generalizations based on specific examples to formulate general rules. Inductive reasoning produces inferences that are valid to a certain degree of credibility or probability. If *x*, *y*, and *z* are men who are mortal, then through induction we may formulate the hypothesis that all men are mortal. Repeated experiments will help to confirm or refute the hypothesis.

In medical practice, inductive reasoning is limited because common events are much easier to perceive than rare ones. Therefore, diagnosis and signs may appear as covariant even though they are not related. These false correlations reduce the quality and reliability of the data.

Abduction

Abductive reasoning, often referred to as the scientific method, is an important part of scientific research. We attempt to establish links between observations such as cause and effect. Hypotheses may help formulate a rule to establish a link between the preceding and subsequent facts (e.g., a diagnosis hypothesis), or they may concern the formulation of a new rule (e.g., a scientific discovery). Supposing the hypothesis is true, deductive reasoning lets us infer new facts that must be confirmed through subsequent examinations or new scientific experiments.

Causal Reasoning

Medical signs and symptoms frequently appear in a particular chronological order, as is the case with infectious or parasitic diseases. *Causal imputation* uses detailed analysis of this chronology and the relationship between the cause and its supposed effects. For example, when trying to attribute a side effect to a drug, we verify:

- that the drug was administered before the appearance of the side effect;
- that the delay before the appearance is compatible with our knowledge of the effect of the drug;

and eventually

- that removing the cause removes the effect (reversibility);
- that, if ethically possible, reintroducing the drug makes the effect re-appear;
- and that the intensity of the effect is proportional to the quantity administered.

Causal reasoning uses abductive or deductive reasoning, depending on the case.

The Steps Involved in Making a Medical Decision

Three basic steps are involved in every medical decision (Figure 4.2).

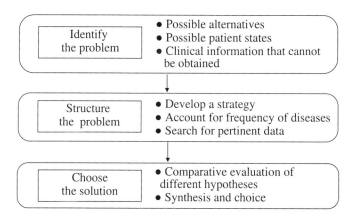

Figure 4.2 : Structure of the decision-making process

Identify the Problem

The first step is to identify the problem, which determines the appropriate area of knowledge. Diagnostic decisions begin with the primary interpretation of clinical data (see the preceding chapter). The clinical technician must select the significant information from among all the initial data (*abstraction*). The identification of pertinent information depends on the experience of the decider. Abductive reasoning is used.

Structure the Problem

The second step is to structure the problem and the clinical information. Several interpretations of the same data or parts of that data are possible. Diagnostic hypotheses are formulated by structuring the information. Reasoning may be deductive (e.g., for a pathognomonic sign), inductive (e.g., diagnosing a transmissive disease in a population of subjects at risk), or abductive.

Choose the Solution

In order to solve a problem, it must often be transformed. Starting with a poorly defined problem — What is the patient's illness? — the physician must arrive at a well-defined problem — Is the patient suffering from disease *x*?

Starting from a number of working hypotheses, the expected signs and symptoms may be obtained by deduction and, if necessary, by the complementary examinations required to obtain them. By induction and/or abduction, the physician may eliminate hypotheses that do not correspond to the observations. The results of complementary examinations may help to reduce the uncertainty over the clinical situation and eliminate hypotheses or solicit new ones.

This process is based on knowledge that has been acquired, memorized, and structured. The physician looks for new diagnostic interpretations when a hypothesis is unsatisfactory or in contradiction with the knowledge he or she already has. This step in the diagnostic process is characterized by cognitive operations that evaluate the interpretations. It requires the clinical technician's active participation in order to control the flow of useful information. The clinical technician must consider the cost of the various strategies.

Uncertainty and Medical Judgment

Medical Judgment

Two clinical technicians confronted with the same situation may use very different decision-making strategies. This is particularly true if we consider the use of specialized and invasive examinations. In fact, a physician's judgments may be represented by Brunswick's general lens model (Figure 4.3). Judgments are based on criteria (*A*, *B*, *C*, etc.) and the relationships that exist on the one hand, between the uncertain situation and the selected criteria and, on the other hand, between the judgment and the criteria. Brunswick stresses that judgments are made in a probabilistic, inexact environment. Any information gathered must be weighed against the environment and the judge's memory when being interpreted, and these elements are combined to reach the final verdict.

The decision-making process lets us

- combine different sources of information that are not statistically independent, in particular redundant clinical and paraclinical information;
- take into account the reliability of the various sources of information;
- consider the predictive value of the various sources of information; and
- bring into play the effects of the task's structure.

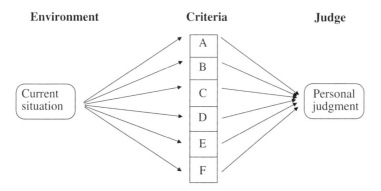

Figure 4.3 : The Brunswick lens model.

Uncertainty and Judgment Bias

Medical judgment may be hindered by the *cognitive bias* that appears throughout the decision-making process:

- When acquiring data, the *order* in which information is provided is a possible source of error, since the first information supplied may dominate the rest.

- Human judgment does not always fully account for *data reliability* (data sources are considered as being perfectly reliable).
- Collecting information is based on *expectations* depending on the context as extrapolated by the decision-maker.
- *Conservatism* is the difficulty of revising opinions, the tendency to favor a particular interpretation, and to rationalize or ignore contrary evidence.
- The *inconsistency* of any judgment represents the contradiction that arises from giving different opinions on identical cases.
- *Justifiability* makes us inclined to apply a rule if we can find a reason to justify it, even if it is not appropriate.

These examples illustrate the difficulty in understanding the decision-making process and its corollary — how decisions are evaluated.

Probability Theory and Decision Analysis

All of the causes for uncertainty discussed previously illustrate the need for a precise scientific framework to represent and manage the problem. Formal decision analysis methods are useful for several reasons:

- They provide a language for expressing and quantifying uncertainty that is more rigorous and less ambiguous than normal language.
- They offer a systematic method for structuring and analyzing problems.
- They help analyze contentious points by identifying differences and specifying their causes.

Probabilities are normally the axiomatic bases of decision theory because they measure the *credibility* of uncertain propositions. Appendix A presents the basic formulas of probability theory.

Comparing Several Diagnostic Hypotheses

Bayes' theorem may be used to evaluate the probabilities of different diagnostic hypotheses. Bayes' formula is reviewed in Appendix A. As signs and symptoms are evaluated (present or absent), the probabilities assigned to each diagnostic are modified, as the example in Figure 4.4 illustrates. In this example, we consider three diagnostic hypotheses (appendicitis, salpingitis, and another diagnosis) and two symptoms (pain in the right lower quadrant,

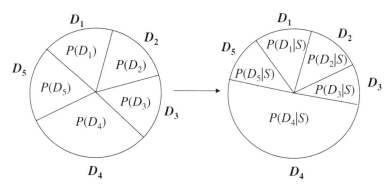

Figure 4.4 : Illustration of Bayes' theorem. Five diagnostics D_i are possible a priori. Knowledge of the sign S modifies the values of the probabilities for each $D_{i.}$

written PRLQ, and pain in the left lower quadrant, written PLLQ) with the following probabilities:

D_i	A priori probability $P(D_i)$	$P(\text{PRLQ}|D_i)$	$P(\text{PLLQ}|D_i)$
Appendicitis	0.10	0.80	0.10
Salpingitis	0.05	0.50	0.50
Other	0.85	0.05	0.05

The *a posteriori* probabilities of the three diagnoses (appendicitis, salpingitis, and other) are calculated for a patient presenting both PRLQ and PLLQ. The calculation first uses the PRLQ symptom, then the PLLQ symptom, knowing that PRLQ is present:

D_i	$PD_i|\text{PRLQ}$	$P(D_i|\text{PRLQ} \wedge \text{PLLQ})$
Appendicitis	0.54	0.35
Salpingitis	0.17	0.55
Other	0.29	0.09

Unfortunately, the difficulties involved in estimating the *a priori* probabilities and conditional probabilities limit the practical use of the Bayes method. We must also make the following hypotheses:

- Diseases are mutually exclusive (a disease may only present one of the D_i diagnoses, as in Figure 4.4).
- The different signs and symptoms involved in the diagnosis are independent.

These two conditions are rarely seen in medical practice.

Evaluating the Benefits of Therapy

Therapy may be curative (e.g., antibiotic treatment or removing a tumor), preventive (e.g., eliminating or reducing a risk factor), palliative (e.g., treating pain) or supportive (e.g., psychological assistance). It is important to be able to estimate the benefits of a given type of therapy for a given patient, as these affect the physician's decision. In practice, these benefits are rarely quantified.

Nonetheless, in some cases these benefits may be evaluated using information supplied by controlled therapeutic tests, whose results may be accessed by querying knowledge bases such as the COCHRANE base. This knowledge base, accessible over the Internet, groups results of thousands of clinical tests (see Chapter 6 and Appendix C).

If P_i represents the risk that a certain event E arises in an intervention group, and P_c represents the risk of that same condition in a control group (P_c is called the *baseline risk*), the ratio of P_i/P_c is called the *relative risk* (RR) associated with the test. RR expresses a measure of the reduction of the risk P_i in the intervention group compared to the baseline risk P_c calculated in the control group. Controlled trials normally provide this measurement. (Sometimes published test results supply the odds ratio (OR). Appendix A provides the formula that transforms OR into RR.)

The RR depends little on the baseline risk. It may therefore be applied to the case of a given patient. If we apply the treatment to the patient, the risk that the event arises will be equal to its own baseline risk P_c multiplied by the relative risk measured in the test. The value of the patient's baseline risk P_c may be estimated from epidemiological data in the literature.

The necessary number of identical subjects that must be treated (NNT, for *Number Needed to Treat*) to avoid event E lets us evaluate the benefits of the therapy. It is calculated as

$$\text{NNT} = \frac{1}{P_c \times (1 - \text{RR})} \tag{4.1}$$

Figure 4.5 illustrates these concepts as applied to the reduction of the risk of death after coronary thrombosis during the ISIS tests [ISIS4 1995]. The percentage of deaths in the control group is 7.8%. For comparable patients, 111 would have to be treated by captopril to avoid one death and 500 with mononitrate [Chatellier 1996].

Drug	Deaths in control group (1)	Deaths in test group (2)	ARR (1)-(2)	RR (2)/(1)	RRR (1-RR)	NNT
Captopril	7.80%	6.90%	0.9%	88.5%	11.5%	111
Mononitrate	7.80%	7.60%	0.2%	97.4%	2.6%	500

Figure 4.5 : Evaluating the benefits of two treatments after coronary thrombosis in the ISIS4 tests. ARR = absolute risk reduction; RR = relative risk; RRR = relative risk reduction; NNT = number needed to treat (see Appendix A)

Decision Analysis

Decision Trees

Medical actions often appear as a series of steps involving decisions: What information should be gathered? Should I carry out further examinations? Should I apply a treatment and, if so, which one? What type of supervision is required? At each step, it is important to consider the benefits and costs of each possible strategy while taking into account knowledge and experience, local capabilities for intervention, and patient preferences.

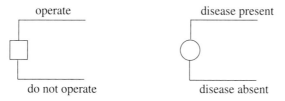

Figure 4.6 : Decision node and contingency node

Decision trees are useful for representing logical sequences and for structuring clinical decision problems. Figure 4.6 presents the two types of nodes that appear in these trees. *Decision nodes*, which are under the control of the decision-maker, are represented by squares. *Contingency nodes*, represented by circles, are not controlled by the decision-maker. The tree presents all the possible strategies, as well as the contingencies that should be considered.

The Concept of Utility

Utilities are quantities used to assign degrees of preference to different solutions and to select the optimal one the *maximum expected utility*. Figure 4.7 illustrates a sample calculation of the expected utility of a given strategy.

A utility may be a probability of survival, a financial risk, or any other function that involves objective or subjective criteria. We must supply the probabilities (the likelihood of the action's potential consequences) and the utilities (the way in which each potential consequence provides a satisfactory solution to the problem). The strategy offering the highest utility is chosen.

Example of Decision Analysis

The tree in Figure 4.8 structures the following clinical problem, borrowed from Weinstein and colleagues [Weinstein 1980]. A 68-year-old diabetic man, wounded on his left foot, has developed an infection that could cause gangrene. Two therapeutic solutions are possible: to amputate or to wait and treat the problem with medication. Medical treatment of the infection could cure the infection but, if ineffective, could require a larger amputation (above the knee) or cause death. Immediate amputation would be below the knee. There is always a risk of death during the operation. What is the best treat-

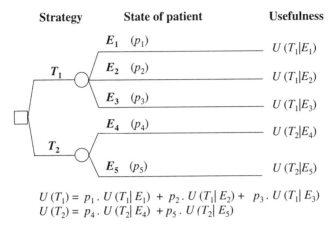

$$U(T_1) = p_1 . U(T_1| E_1) + p_2 . U(T_1| E_2) + p_3 . U(T_1| E_3)$$
$$U(T_2) = p_4 . U(T_2| E_4) + p_5 . U(T_2| E_5)$$

Figure 4.7 : Calculating the utility of a strategy. The preferred strategy is
the one that offers the highest utility

ment? Based on the utilities provided and the probabilities associated with
each possibility, immediate amputation was the selected strategy.

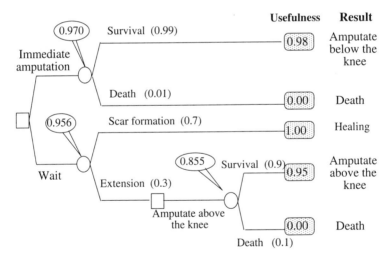

Figure 4.8 : Decision tree from [Weinstein 1980]. Utilities have been set
subjectively on a scale of 0 to 1

Symbolic Reasoning and Expert Systems

Over the last 15 years, decision support systems have been developed by
tackling problems in the most general way possible. Research has been

directed especially toward solving problems for which no algorithmic solution exists. This method has led researchers to suggest means for representing and using symbolic and declarative knowledge that enriches and complements numerical and algorithmic methods. The methods and techniques of *artificial intelligence* (AI) have provided a privileged framework for cognitive research and have led to the development of expert systems. These numerous developments are now used in all medical specialties.

Knowledge Representation

Several types of knowledge are required for symbolic reasoning: anatomical, pathological, epidemiological, taxonomic (in particular, concerning the classification of patients), pharmacological, and therapeutic. On the cognitive level, we may define two principal knowledge models:

1. The empirical model. *Empirical knowledge* concerns the associations between diseases and symptoms. They may be provided by an expert or derived from the analysis of a database.

2. Models based on *physiological and pathological knowledge*. This type of knowledge, when available, lets us employ reasoning that describes the mechanisms involved in morbid processes. Explanations supplied by causal knowledge are more easily understood by a user who did not participate in the development of the decision-support system.

Two major formal systems for representing knowledge are used: production rules and frames.

Production Rules

These indicate that if the conditions or premises are met, the conclusions may be affirmed. The conclusions may be a diagnostic hypothesis or an action (additional tests, indication of a treatment, etc.). The general form for such rules is

IF *<conditions>* THEN *<conclusions>*.

Figure 4.9 illustrates one of the hundreds of production rules in the MYCIN expert system, developed by experts in infectious diseases. MYCIN

IF:	The grain stain of the organism is gram-negative The morphology of the organism is rod The patient is at risk
THEN:	Suggest (credibility = 0.6) that the infecting agent is *Pseudomonas*

Figure 4.9 : Sample production rule from the MYCIN expert system

applies rules by combining the degree of credibility assigned to each rule. The impact of an inference on the decision may be modified by a *credibility factor* (CF) between −1 and 1. The closer the CF is to 1, the more likely the conclusion (Figure 4.9). Negative values express the negation of the conclusion in the same way. Decision-support systems developed by MYCIN take into account information concerning the patient, and the knowledge of the culture involved, isolated organisms, and the drugs administered [Shortliffe 1976].

Arden syntax is a proposed standard for the representation of production rules, designed after a working seminar at the Arden Homestead, NY, in 1989 [Clayton 1989]. Rules are represented in structured *Medical Logic Modules* (MLM) with the idea of reuse from one institution to the other [Hripcsak 1994].

Frames

Structured objects or *frames* let us describe complex medical concepts by specifying their characteristics and the means for evaluating them [Minsky 1975, Pauker 1976]. Figure 4.10 provides an example of this representation.

NAME: Acute glomerulonephritis	
Triggered by	facial edema, not painful, not erythematous, symmetrical, etc.
Confirmed by	malaise, asthenia, anorexia, etc.
Caused by	recent streptococci infection
Causes	sodium retention, acute hypertension, nephrotic syndrome, etc.
Complications	acute kidney failure
Differential diagnostic	(**If** chronic high blood pressure **then** chronic glomerulonephritis) (**If** recurrent edema **then** nephrotic syndrome)

Figure 4.10 : Example of a medical concept represented by a structured object: a fragment of the description of acute glomerulonephritis

Using Knowledge

The use of knowledge depends to a large extent on the method used for representing knowledge and the chosen strategy. For didactic reasons, we will present the classical strategies used in systems based on production rules.

Backward Chaining in Production Systems

The system creates all possible paths leading to each possible conclusion. Paths are built using rules of knowledge. With the *backward chaining* search strategy, also known as *goal-oriented* strategy, the system uses all the rules leading to a given goal (e.g., *G* in Figure 4.11). To affirm the goal, rules are used one after another. The use of all rules leading to a given goal can be represented in the form of a AND/OR tree.

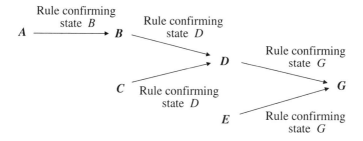

Figure 4.11 : Diagram of an AND/OR tree

In systems with weighted conclusions, credibility factors are created using various models. In MYCIN, for example, the credibility of the conclusion for a premise such as IF *A* THEN *B* is calculated using the following formula:

$$\mathrm{CF}(C) = \partial \cdot \min((\mathrm{CF})(A), \mathrm{CF}(B)) \qquad (4.2)$$

where ∂ is the credibility factor of the rule provided by the expert and $\min(\mathrm{CF}(A), \mathrm{CF}(B))$ is the smaller of $\mathrm{CF}(A)$ and $\mathrm{CF}(B)$. Figure 4.12 presents the rules for combining credibility factors in MYCIN.

Figure 4.13 is a diagram of an AND/OR tree developed by MYCIN. Outlined figures are the results of the formulas from Figure 4.12. These formulas show that certainties are always reinforced in MYCIN [Shortliffe 1976]. In order to limit the effects of this reinforcement mechanism, MYCIN uses simple heuristics. If a node in the AND/OR tree is assigned a credibility with absolute value less than 0.2, it is not considered in future calculations. This is the case of the last node in Figure 4.13, with credibility 0.1. The node at the top of this tree represents a conclusion with credibility as calculated by the system of 0.24.

In systems with weighted conclusions, credibility factors are created using different models. The backward chaining strategy is even more efficient when the selected goal is relevant.

Forward Chaining in Production Systems

With the forward chaining strategy, also known as the data-oriented strategy, the system does not propose goals to be confirmed. It transforms all available information into knowledge rules and attempts to deduct everything that can be deduced.

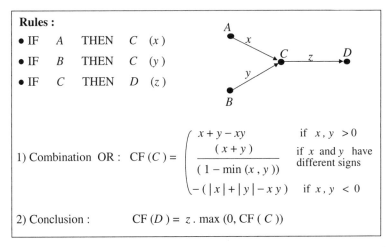

Figure 4.12 : Combination of credibility factors (CF) in MYCIN. x, y and z are the CF of the conclusions of rules supplied by the expert

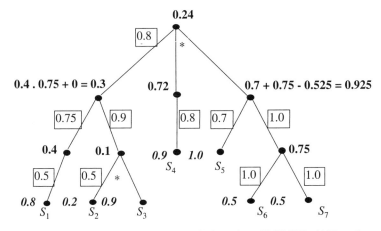

Figure 4.13 : AND/OR tree created by all the rules of MYCIN. AND nodes are marked with a star. The S_i are the signs to be sought in the patient. Outlined numbers rate the credibility of the user for each sign. The CF supplied by the expert (CF of rules) are framed

The data-oriented strategy considers all new information in its reasoning but is exposed to the risks of *combinatory explosions* — the number of deductions may be very high, but they are not relevant to the problem.

Mixed Strategies

Forward and backward chaining may be combined in production rules. For example, given that state *A* is true in the tree in Figure 4.11, we can execute forward chaining going from rule *A* towards *B*, then from *B* to *D*. Using backward chaining, we may attempt to confirm *D* by verifying state *C*, then eventually by executing forward chaining to go towards *G*, and so forth.

Learning

Reasoning and decision-making require the preliminary acquisition and use of knowledge. Learning is of interest for computer scientists in order to develop decision-support systems. A learning system is defined in the Robert dictionary [Robert 1994] as "a system capable of modifying its future answers as a function of past experience".

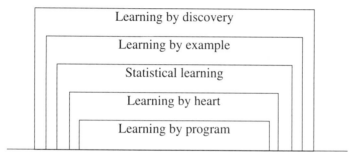

Figure 4.14 : Different types of learning (adapted from [Laurière 1987])

Given the theoretical and practical interest of these systems, it is useful to analyze the various components of learning. Jean-Louis Laurière [Laurière 1987] proposes the following classification (Figure 4.14):

- *Programmed learning*: This corresponds to all current programs where a code controls what must be done. This is the case for robots precisely executing prerecorded commands.
- *Learning "by heart"*: All situations have been memorized. The system must find and apply the behavior corresponding to the situation.
- *Statistical learning*: The system only retains a classification of the situations based on the greatest number of cases.
- *Learning by example*: The system must be able to generalize. It must abstract the knowledge required to solve similar cases from examples. It uses inductive reasoning.
- *Learning by discovery*: The system uses inductive and/or abductive methods. It must be able to create new hypotheses and new concepts.

Discussion and Conclusion

Medical decisions involve very complex processes that are neither clearly
defined nor easily reproduced on computers. If the methods for representing
knowledge and reasoning can answer questions such as "How should I treat a
given patient's disease on a given day?", total patient care goes beyond available resources. Several types of knowledge must be taken into account, representing considerable volumes of information. Problems remain to be
solved concerning the use of different types of knowledge and the integration
and evaluation of expert systems in medical information systems. They are
discussed in Chapter 12.

Exercises

- *List some of the principles of medical reasoning.*
- *What are the main steps in medical decision-making?*
- *List a few biases in judgment.*
- *What is the principle of decision analysis?*
- *Describe the reasoning principles used in expert systems based on pro-
  duction rules.*
- *List a few types of learning.*

5

Medical Language and Classification Systems

Introduction

Medical language uses an extremely rich and difficult vocabulary. The terms employed are often vague and imprecise and are seldom rigorously defined. The same disease may be known under several names or expressions, known as synonymy. Inversely, a single term may have several meanings according to the speaker and the context, known as polysemy.

This situation does not prevent health-care personnel from communicating, but it does considerably complicate the use of computers in the practice of medicine and medical research. As a result, ambiguities must be resolved and vocabulary standardized in order to collect information for epidemiology, public health, clinical research, documentation, or medical decision-making. This is usually achieved by creating classifications and coding systems.

Coding and Classifications

Although they are not synonyms, the words nomenclature, dictionary, thesaurus, classification, and codification are sometimes incorrectly treated as such. The American Heritage Dictionary of the English Language provides the following definitions:

- *Dictionary:* "A reference book containing an alphabetical list of words, with information given for each word, usually including meaning, pronunciation, and etymology".
- *Nomenclature:* "1. A system of names used in an art or a science: the nomenclature of mineralogy. 2. The procedure of assigning names to the kinds and groups of organisms listed in a taxonomic classification: the rules of nomenclature in botany".
- *Thesaurus*: "1. A book of synonyms, often including related and contrasting words and antonyms. 2. A book of selected words or concepts, such as a specialized vocabulary of a particular field, as of medicine or music."

- *Classification:* "1. The act or result of classifying. 2. A category or class. 3. The systematic grouping of organisms into categories on the basis of evolutionary or structural relationships between them; taxonomy." In biology, organisms have long been classified into kingdoms, subkingdoms or phyla, classes, orders, families, tribes, races, species, subspecies, varieties, and forms.
- *Catalog:* "A list or itemized display, as of titles, course offerings, or articles for exhibition or sale, usually including descriptive information or illustrations."
- *Codifying:* "To reduce to a code." Codes are usually numeric or alphanumeric.

Note the difference in use of a dictionary and a thesaurus: dictionaries are usually consulted when the syntax of the word is known but not its meaning. A thesaurus or a classification system is used when we know what we want to say but not how to express it in a standardized vocabulary.

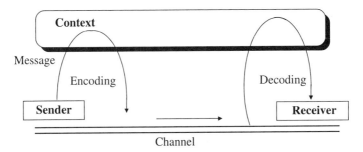

Figure 5.1 : Communicating information

Figure 5.1 illustrates the mechanisms for communicating information using messages. Communication is successful only if the sender and the receiver know both the language (code) and the context. Notice the importance of the latter, which must be identical for both parties.

Whenever possible, the codification should be one-to-one: only one term should exist for a given object, and each term should describe only one object. There is no ambiguity through polysemy or homonymy. These conditions are imperative for successful research and for avoiding impertinent or false answers.

Classifications provide a useful framework for a systematic representation and codification of medical concepts. *Monoaxial classifications* form a hierarchy of terms based on a common root (Figure 5.2). The first-level classes are the principal classes. They must cover the entire sphere. Any object in the sphere belongs to one and only one class. The division must obey a criterion that is applied to all the items in the parent class, while successive criteria are listed in decreasing order of importance. Semantic links within a hierarchy may concern adherence to a class (*is–a* links) or partitioning (*part–of* links). The most commonly used example of monoaxial hierarchical classifications

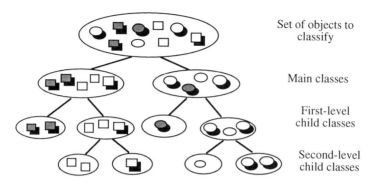

Set of objects to
classify

Main classes

First-level
child classes

Second-level
child classes

Figure 5.2 : Hierarchical classification

is the *International Classification of Diseases* (ICD), published by the World
Health Organization (ICD-9) and its clinical adaptation (ICD-9-CM) [ICD-
9-CM 1994].

Multiaxial or multifaceted classifications combine terms belonging to different classes that themselves may be organized in a hierarchy. SNOMED is
an example of this type of classification [Coté 1993]. This juxtaposition of
terms from different categories is nevertheless insufficient to express the
wealth of semantic links that may exist between medical terms (such as the
active and passive forms of verbs like *to be, to have, to cause, to treat, to
complicate*, etc.). These links or *connectors* are detailed in classifications
systems such as the UMLS [McCray 1989]. They roughly correspond to verb
groups in natural language (e.g., *is a, treats, is treated by, causes, is caused
by*, etc.), as illustrated in Figure 5.3.

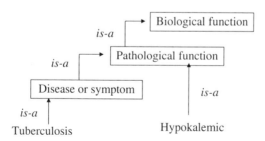

Figure 5.3 : Classification and semantic links between medical terms

Finally, it may be useful to add *modifiers* that perform the role of adjec-
tives in natural language to the semantic fields of the classification (the nom-
inal groups) and the connectors (the verbs). These modifiers may, for
example, indicate the suspected or confirmed degree of certainty, or the
intensity or the increasing evolution of an assertion.

Examples of Classifications

Medical information systems use several vocabularies and lists of medical terms. Some are used on an international level, while others have been defined according to the needs of one or several hospital departments. We will briefly present a few of these systems, although none of them is entirely satisfactory. Some of the medical entities in such a classification will seem insufficiently detailed to some specialists or too complex to use. In any case, it is useful to establish rules for translating from one system to another.

Clinical Classifications

International Classifications of Diseases

The *International Classification of Diseases* (ICD) was designed for world-wide use. Its historical origins are briefly described in Figure 5.4. Regular revisions of this classification appear as of 1900 and, as of 1946, the WHO assumed responsibility for the ICD.

1853	W. Farr (1807–1883) Standard nomenclature for causes of death
1893	J. Bertillon (1851–1922) New classification for causes of death
1946	WHO International Statistical Classification of Diseases, Trauma and Causes of Death
1975	Ninth revision (ICD-9)
1979	Clinical Modification (ICD-9-CM, HCIMO)
1992	International Statistical Classification of Diseases and Related Health Problems (ICD-10)

Figure 5.4 : History of the International Classification of Diseases (ICD)

The ninth revision, known as ICD-9, dates from 1975 [OMS 1977]. Very widespread today, it is based on the two following major classifications principles:

- Diseases are divided into categories with a common characteristic. This characteristic may be etiological (e.g., infectious diseases), may refer to a particular system (e.g., cardiovascular or pulmonary diseases), or may designate the morbid process (e.g., neoplastic diseases) (Figure 5.5).
- Each category is sub-divided into hierarchical levels that enable a precise diagnosis.
- Every entry in the classification includes a four-digit hierarchical code with an optional fifth digit in some cases:

ICD-9 is a compromise between classifications based on etiology, anatomical locations, and details of appearance. It does not describe how a given disease occurs nor does it codify the clinical details for a given patient. Given its initial objective, the notions of time (recurrent, progressively worsens, etc.) and of physiology-pathology (respiratory alcalosis, bronchial hyperreactivity, etc.) are practically absent from ICD-9. A clinical modification was proposed as of 1977 in the United States under the name of ICD-9-CM, and annual updates are published by the Health Care Financing Administration (HCFA) [ICD-9-CM 1994]. The modifications mainly concern the addition of one or two digits to the ICD-9 codes. Since 1989, the reimbursement of Medicare expenses requires the respect of ICD-9-CM codification. The National Center for Health Statistics (NCHS) and the HCFA are the two U.S. governmental agencies responsible for overseeing all changes to the ICD-9-CM.

I	Infectious and parasitic diseases
II	Neoplasms
III	Endocrine, nutritional and metabolic diseases, and immunity disorders
IV	Diseases of the blood and blood-forming organs
V	Mental disorders
VI	Diseases of the nervous system and sense organs
VII	Diseases of the circulatory system
VIII	Diseases of the respiratory system
IX	Diseases of the digestive system
X	Diseases of the genitourinary system
XI	Complications of pregnancy, childbirth and the puerperium
XII	Diseases of the skin and subcutaneous tissue
XIII	Diseases of the musculoskeletal system and connective tissue
XIV	Congenital abnormalities
XV	Certain conditions originating in the perinatal period
XVI	Symptoms, signs and ill-defined conditions
XVII	Injury and poisoning
Supplementary Classifications	
E	External causes of injury and poisoning
III	Factors influencing health status and contact with health services

Figure 5.5 : The categories of ICD-9

The latest revision, the ICD-10, was published in 1992 (Figure 5.4) [ICD-10 1992]. It takes into account recent experience, corrects a few deficiencies of the previous versions, and offers a new structure. Clearly, it is not possible for a single classification system to meet all needs for more or less detailed classifications that may be useful in different circumstances. The tenth revision proposes to define a "family of classifications of diseases and related health classifications," of which the ICD-10 is the kernel.

Figure 5.6 lists the categories that structure the ICD-10. The ICD-10 uses an alphanumeric code with one letter followed by two digits for three-character categories or three digits for four-character categories. Important new features have been included, such as, at the end of certain chapters, the creation of categories concerning post-therapeutic problems.

I	Certain infectious and parasitic diseases
II	Neoplasms
III	Diseases of the blood and blood-forming organs and certain disorders involving the immune mechanism
IV	Endocrine, nutritional and metabolic diseases
V	Mental and behavioral disorders
VI	Diseases of the nervous system
VII	Diseases of the eye and adnexa
VIII	Diseases of the ear and mastoid process
IX	Diseases of the circulatory system
X	Diseases of the respiratory system
XI	Diseases of the digestive system
XII	Diseases of the skin and subcutaneous tissue
XIII	Diseases of the musculoskeletal system and connective tissue
XIV	Diseases of the genitourinary system
XV	Pregnancy, childbirth and the puerperium
XVI	Certain conditions originating in the perinatal period
XVII	Congenital malformations, deformations and chromosomal abnormalities
XVIII	Symptoms, sign and abnormal clinical and laboratory findings, not elsewhere classified
XIX	Injury, poisoning and certain other consequences of external causes
XX	External causes of morbidity and mortality
XXI	Factors influencing health status and contact with health services
Supplementary Classifications	
M	Morphology of neoplasms

Figure 5.6 : The categories of ICD-10

Figure 5.7 presents an extract of the list of three-character diseases with examples of links with other terms.

L93	Lupus erythematosus
	Excludes: lupus:
	         • exedens (A18.4)
	         • vulgaris (A18.4)
	         scleroderma (M34.–)
	         systematic lupus erythematosus (M32.–)
	Use additional external cause code (Chapter XX), id desired, to identify drug, if drug-induced.

L93.0	Discoid lupus erythematosus Lupus erythematosus NOS
L93.1	Subacute cutaneous lupus erythematosus

Figure 5.7 : Detail of the International Classification of Diseases (ICD-10)

A clinical modification of ICD-10 (ICD-10-CM) for morbidity purposes is currently developed by the NCHS.

Read Codes

The Read Codes, developed in Great Britain, are a comprehensive list of terms intended for use by all healthcare professionals to describe the care and treatment of their patients. They enable the capture and retrieval of patient centred information in natural clinical language within computer systems.

The Read Codes are used by a significant proportion of family practitioners within the UK, to record details about patient care and for the business needs of the practice. Read Codes and their maintenance by the NHS Centre for Coding and Classification. Version 3 terms are provided, where appropriate, with validated cross-references to ICD-9, ICD-10 and OPCS-4 (*Office of Population Censuses and Surveys Classification of Surgical Operations and Procedures,* 4th revision).

B.... *Neoplasms*
   B1... *Malignant neoplasm of digestive organs*
     B15. *Malignant neoplasm of liver*
             B150. *Primary malignant neoplasm of liver*
             B150 *Hepatoblastoma of liver*

Figure 5.8 : Detail of the Read Codes

The NANDA Classification of Nursing Diagnoses

The NANDA classification is a set of nursing diagnoses adopted by the *North American Nursing Diagnosis Association* (NANDA). NANDA nursing diagnoses describe patients' reactions to the disease. They are organized around nine "Human Response Patterns":

1. Exchanging
2. Communicating
3. Relating
4. Valuing
5. Choosing
6. Moving
7. Perceiving
8. Knowing
9. Feeling

Within each pattern, NANDA lists one to four subcategories. For example, under Exchanging, 1.3.2 is "altered urinary elimination", and 1.3.2.1.3 is "urge incontinence".

Classification of Treatments and Procedures

The classification of treatments and procedures varies considerably from country to country, in particular due to the multiplicity of systems concerning the reimbursement and/or the evaluation of resources used (see Chapter 14).

Classification of Procedures in the ICD-9-CM

In parallel with the development of the CPT, a classification of procedures for the ICD-9-CM was created based on a working document of the WHO, published on the occasion of the ninth revision under the title "*ICD-9, Classification of Procedures in Medicine, Fascicle V, Surgical Procedures*". The classification, organized in a hierarchical manner (Fig. 5.9), includes four digits, of which two are decimal numbers [ICD-9-CM 1994].

35–39 Operations on the cardiovascular system
35 Operations on valves and septa of heart
> Includes: sternotomy, thoractomy as operative approach
> Code also cardiopulmonary bypass (39.61)

35.0 Closed heart valvotomy
> | Excludes: | percutaneous (balloon) valvuloplasty (35.96)
> 35.00 Closed heart valvotomy, unspecified valve
> 35.01 Closed heart valvotomy, aortic valve
> 35.02 Closed heart valvotomy, mitral valve
> ...

35.1 Open heart valvuloplasty without replacement
...
35.2 Replacement of heart valve

Figure 5.9 : Example of the classification of procedures in ICD-9-CM

Current Procedural Terminology

In the United States, the CPT *(Current Procedural Terminology)* classification was developed under the aegis of the American Medical Association [AMA 1999]. The first version was published in 1966, and the fourth edition, known as CPT 4, has been the basis for codification of procedures, called the *Health Care Common Procedure Coding System* (HCPCS), of the HCFA.

Urinary System	
Kidney	
Incision	
	(For retroperitoneal exploration, abscess, tumor, or cyst, see 49010, 49060, 49200, 49201)
50010	Renal exploration, not necessitating other specific procedures
50020	Drainage of perirenal or renal abscess (separate procedure)
50040	Nephrostomy, nephrotomy with drainage
50045	Nephrotomy with exploration
	(For renal endoscopy performed in conjunction with this procedure, see 50570-50580)

Figure 5.10 : Extract of the Current Procedural Terminology (CPT 4)

The CADAM Catalog of Medical Procedures

The catalog of medical procedures (*Catalogue Des Actes Médicaux,* or CDAM) was prepared by the French Ministry of Health to implement the reform of public hospital finances and the program for "medicalizing" the information system (*Programme de Médicalisation du Système d'Information,* or PMSI), a system for tracking medical activity (see Chapter 14). It is very close to the HCIMO concerning the treatments that are defined and encoded, but unfortunately does not include a hierarchical structure. It is subdivided into seven fields represented by Greek letters (Figure 5.10).

ALPHA (AL)	Diagnostic and therapeutic treatments
BETA (BE)	Anesthesiology
GAMMA (GA)	Imaging
MU (MU)	Radiotherapy
RHO (RH)	Morphology
TAU (TO)	Biology
OMEGA (OM)	Reanimation

Figure 5.11 : Catalog of medical treatments (CDAM)

The treatment code contains four characters (one letter and three numbers). Each treatment is assigned a three-digit relative cost index *(Index de coût Relatif,* or ICR*),* the medical domain in which it is located, and a reference. Major treatments (those consuming significant resources) are indicated by the letter X. The ICR helps to quantify the economic consequences of the treatment, as in the following example:

"Appendectomy for acute appendicitis: L260   050   AL   X"

A study is currently under way to create a single NGAP-CDAM nomenclature that would meet the specific analytical requirements of the healthcare organizations promoting these two nomenclatures.

LOINC Codes

The LOINC™ (*Logical Observation Identifiers, Names and Codes*) database provides a set of universal names and ID codes for identifying laboratory and clinical observations. The LOINC codes are not intended to transmit all possible information about a test. They are mainly intended to identify the test results. Other fields in a message are required to transmit the identity of the source laboratory and the very detailed information on the specimen.

Multidomain Classifications

SNOMED Nomenclature

The SNOMED (*Systematized Nomenclature of Medicine*) nomenclature is an example of a multi-axial classification, developed by North American pathologists and extended from the SNOP (*Systematic Nomenclature of*

Pathology). The third edition, called *SNOMED International*, contains more than 200,000 terms used in medical and veterinary practice [Côté 1993] (Figure 5.12).

	ICD-10	**SNOMED-International**
Structure	Multi-axial	Hierarchical, multiaxial (linked axes)
Code format	A99.9	T,M,F,L,C,A,J,S,D,P,G 99999[9]
A code represents	A group of terms	A concept
Number of entries	80,000 (index included)	130,000 records
Contents	Diagnoses, symptoms, abnormal laboratory results, wounds and poisoning, external causes of death and morbidity, factors influencing the state of health	Topography, etiology, morphology, organisms, drugs and medications, diseases, procedures, occupations, general modifiers, physical agents, social context

Figure 5.12 : Comparison of CIM-10 and SNOMED-International

SNOMED is organized around 11 main axes called *modules*, designated by the following letters:

- T for *topography*, which describes the parts of the body, organs, and regions (12,385 records).
- M for *morphology*, which presents congenital or acquired modifications of the anatomy, cells, or organs. This module includes the morphological nomenclature of tumors described in the International Classification of Diseases for Oncology (ICD-O) which appeared in 1990 (4,991 records).

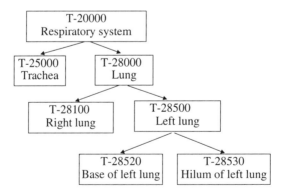

Figure 5.13 : Hierarchical organization of the topography axis in SNOMED international

- F for *function*, which describes the terms of physiopathology and the terms used to described both normal and pathological states and processes (16,352 records).
- L for *living organisms*, a classification of animals and plants that are essentially pathogens or carriers of disease (25,265 records).
- C for *chemicals, drugs and biological products*, presenting the classes of drugs and medication as well as chemical products and plant extracts (14,075 records).
- A for *physical agents, forces and activities*, which compiles a list of activities and instruments associated with diseases or traumas (1,355 records).
- J for *occupation*, which is used to codify professional activities according to a classification developed by the International Labour Office (ILO) (1,886 records).
- S for *social context*, which offers a list of social situations that are interesting from a medical standpoint (433 records).
- D for *disease*, which describes the diseases and combinations of signs and symptoms (syndromes and complex diseases). It also provides a correspondence with the diagnostic terms from the ICD-9-CM (28,622 records).
- P for *procedure*, which presents administrative, diagnostic, and therapeutic activities used to prevent or treat diseases (approximately 25,000 records).
- G for *general linkage/ modifiers*, which establishes a list of terms used to qualify and link together the terms of the various modules (1,176 records).The elements within each axis are organized in a hierarchical structure, as shown in Figure 5.13, for the topography of pulmonary locations.

Codes are created by juxtaposing the codes belonging to the various classifications, as shown in Figure 5.14 which represents the concept of pulmonary tuberculosis.

T	+	M	+	E	+	F	+	D
Lung		Granuloma		*M. tuberculosis*		Fever		Tuberculosis
T-2800		M-44060		E-2001		F-03003		D-0188

Figure 5.14 : Sample SNOMED codification

SNOMED has been used successfully on an international basis in areas such as anatomy-pathology and radiology. It has been translated into several languages. Recent development concern the use of SNOMED as a reference terminology for health care [Spackman 1997]. Concepts included in the coming version named SNOMED RT include data relating to the causes and symptoms of diseases, the treatment of patients, and the outcome of the overall health care process. Proposed changes allow SNOMED RT to represent multiple types of hierarchies (e.g., is-a, part-of) and to make the types fully explicit [Spackman 1997].

MeSH Thesaurus

The MeSH (*Medical Subject Headings*) thesaurus was designed in the early 1960s by the *National Library of Medicine* (NLM) in Bethesda, Maryland, to automatically create the INDEX MEDICUS, a directory of major scientific publications [MeSH 1998] (see Chapter 6).

A	Anatomy
B	Organisms
C	Diseases
D	Drugs and chemical products
E	Analytical, diagnostic, and therapeutic techniques and equipment
F	Psychiatry and psychology
G	Biological sciences
H	Physical sciences
I	Anthropology, education, sociology, and social phenomena
J	Technology, industry, agriculture, and food
K	Humanities
L	Information sciences and communication
M	Named groups
N	Health
Z	Geographical names

Figure 5.15 : The MeSH classification

The 1999 edition of MeSH includes more than 19,000 main headings, 100,000 supplementary chemicals, and an entry vocabulary of over 250,000 terms. The MeSH thesaurus is continually updated and covers most areas of health (Figure 5.15). It has been translated into several languages including German, Spanish, French, and Portuguese.

A descriptor is an expression chosen from a set of terms judged as equivalent for unambiguously representing a single concept. It may be in a simple format (e.g., a single term, such as: "Greenland") or composed of several terms (e.g., a precoordinated descriptor, such as: "pregnancy with complications").

Each descriptor is assigned an alphanumeric code that describes the position of the term in one or several hierarchies of terms. A hierarchical tree may have up to seven levels. Figure 5.16 illustrates the hierarchical structure of the MeSH vocabulary. Descriptors may be major or minor. They are described in detail in the alphabetical MeSH that makes up the actual thesaurus (Figure 5.16). The descriptors are written in uppercase letters in the thesaurus. The major descriptors (e.g., GENETIC MARKERS) represent key points. Minor descriptors (e.g., CHROMOSOME MAPPING) refer to the major descriptors. Equivalences and synonymous relationships are indicated by the verb *see* placed between a term and a descriptor, and by the letter *X* between a descriptor and a term. Major descriptors that are closely related are indicated by the expressions *see related* and *XR*. Hierarchical relationships between major and minor descriptors are indicated by the expression *see under* and its inverse by the characters *XU*.

```
CORONARY VESSELS, DISEASES C14.280.211
  ANGINA                     C14.280.211.198
    PRINZMETAL'S ANGINA      C14.280.211.198.955  C14.280.211
    UNSTABLE ANGINA          C14.280.211.198.970
  CORONARY ANEURYSM          C14.280.211.205      C14.907.55
  ARTERIOSCLEROSIS           C14.280.211.210      C14.907.137
  CORONARY THROMBOSIS        C14.280.211.212      C14.907.854
  CORONARY SPASM                                  C14.280.211.215
```

Figure 5.16 : The hierarchical structure of the MesH system

MeSH provides access to the INDEX MEDICUS and the MEDLINE database, which contains several hundred thousand bibliographical references (see Chapter 6).

```
GENETIC MARKERS
      D24.185.101.387              G5.735.450
usually NIM; IM GEN only; coord with specific genetic feature (IM) if
pertinent; only /anal /blood-csf-urine
89; was GENETIC MARKER  1980-88
use GENETIC MARKERS to search GENETIC MARKER back thru 1980
see related
      CHROMOSOME MAPPING
X     CHROMOSOME MARKERS
X     DNA MARKERS
X     MARKERS, DNA
X     MARKERS,  GENETIC

GENETIC  SCREENING
      E1.563.390                   E5.318.370.580.120
      G3.850.520.610.580.120       N1.224.458.527.125
      N2.421.143.827.233.443.125
only /instrum /methods /trends /vet
78
see related
      HETEROZYGOTE DETECTION

GENETIC  TECHNICS
      E5.393+
do not use \man \methods \supply  /util      CATALOG: do not use  73
XR    GENETIC COUNSELING
```

Figure 5.17 : The structure of the alphabetical MeSH

The Unified Medical Language System

The *Unified Medical Language System* (UMLS) project, developed since 1986 by the National Library of Medicine in Bethesda, Maryland, attempts to establish a conceptual link between the user's requirements for a certain piece of information and different sources of information such as databases on medical literature, medical record management systems, or knowledge bases (Figure 5.17). Since a single concept may be expressed in different ways through these sources, it is very important to determine which ones contain pertinent information for a given query [McCray 1989, Lindberg 1993, Campbell 1998].

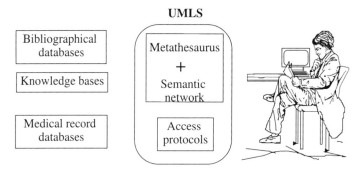

Figure 5.18 : The UMLS Approach

The knowledge of UMLS is contained in the metathesaurus, the UMLS's semantic network, the descriptions of the sources of information called the *Information Source Map,* and the lexicon [UMLS 1996]. The 1998 version of the metathesaurus contains approximately 480,000 concepts and more than 1,000,000 different concept names. It groups together (hence the prefix meta) terms from about 40 biomedical vocabularies and classifications including MeSH 99 (394,300 strings), READ Codes 98 (340,000 strings), SNOMED 3.5 (164,200 strings), LOINC 97 (40,500), ICD-9-CM (19,700), ICD-10 (13,500 terms), HCPCS (Healthcare Financing Administration Common Procedure Coding System) 99 (11,400 strings), the DSM-IV (*Diagnostic and Statistical Manual of Mental Disorders, 4th Edition*), the CPT 4 classification *(Current Procedural Terminology)*, as well as concepts used in knowledge bases such as PDQ, DXPLAIN, and QMR or selected medical record management systems such as COSTAR.

The *semantic network* contains the relationships between certain semantic categories. For example, "virus" *may–cause* "disease or syndrome". Figure 5.19 presents a simplified example of the semantic network.

The *information source map* describes the databases, their contents, their vocabularies, their level of coverage, and the conditions for access.

The *specialist lexicon* contains linguistic information needed by natural language processing (NLP) systems (e.g., syntactic, morphological, and gra-

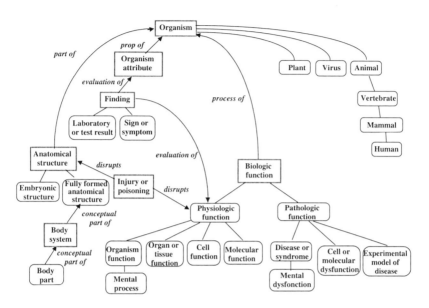

Figure 5.19 : The semantic network of the UMLS language (adapted from
UMLS 1995, NIH/NLM, 6th experimental edition, April 1995)

phemic information). It includes biomedical and general English terms
[McCray 1998].

Discussion and Conclusion

The quality of a classification may be judged by its sensitivity and specificity
when replying to queries made to databases using it. The sensitivity and
specificity depend on the following elements:

- *Completeness:* A complete description of the medical field is very difficult to achieve.
- *Nonambiguity:* The terms must refer to only one concept. If a term is
  ambiguous, at least two different types of data are stored under the same
  term, which affects the specificity of the replies.
- *Nonredundancy:* Each concept should only be expressed in one way. If
  two terms refer to the same concept, the sensitivity of the replies to database queries will be reduced.
- *Synonyms:* The ability to manage synonyms is important. It should be
  distinguished from redundancy, which must be avoided. Synonyms are
  authorized intermediate terms that refer to a unique term (the internal
  code) used to encode, index, and find the useful information.

- *Explicit relationships:* When the types of relationships between terms in a nomenclature are not clear, the quality of the replies to queries will suffer. *Is–a, is–part–of, causes, associated–with, equivalent–to, is–in* are the most common relationships. If we want to query a database to find the pulmonary diseases of a patient, we will locate all terms with an *is–a* relationship to the concept of "pulmonary disease".

The table in Figure 5.19 reviews the properties of four representative classifications.

	ICD-10	SNOMED	MeSH	UMLS
Complete	No	Yes	Yes	Yes
Unambiguous	No	Yes	No	Yes
Non redundant	Yes	No	Yes	Yes
Synonyms	Yes	Yes	Yes	Yes
Explicit relations	Yes	Yes	Yes	Yes

Figure 5.20 : Comparing different classifications

Since the control of codifications is not always guaranteed, *transcoding* (going from one classification to another) is usually difficult. The problems involved in transcoding are another reason to carefully choose a codification system. It is generally best to find the most widespread and widely used classification, updated regularly by a competent, recognized international organization.

Exercises

- *Define a dictionary, a thesaurus, a classification, a nomenclature, and a catalog.*
- *Describe the principle of encoding and decoding medical information.*
- *Describe the organizational principles and structure of the International Classification of Diseases (ICD).*
- *Describe the methods for classifying procedures and the problems involved.*
- *Describe the organizational principles and structure of SNOMED.*
- *Describe the organizational principles and structure of the MeSH language.*
- *Describe the organizational principles and structure of the UMLS language.*

6

Documentation Systems and Information Databases

Introduction

The number of cataloged medical periodicals is increasing exponentially, doubling approximately every 10 to 15 years, and today surpasses 20,000. There are more than 250,000 individualized medical concepts in the UMLS metathesaurus (see Chapter 5). Unfortunately, the time physicians and researchers are able to devote to reading scientific texts is not expandable. Given this situation, it is easy to imagine the need to use automatic systems to access medical knowledge.

Documentation systems are very diverse. Some systems, such as bibliographic databases, are used as information indexes. They do not contain all the desired and useful information but only the means to access this information. Others try to directly provide the end-user with the required information. Full text databases and knowledge banks enter in this category. In the first case, information is updated essentially by adding new references. In the second case, updates are made through additions and corrections because medical knowledge is in a state of permanent evolution.

Technical Infrastructure

Document management systems and information and knowledge bases are stored on data servers accessible from the desktop via communication networks (Figure 6.1).

Workstations

The workstation may be a simple visual display unit, a microcomputer, or a high-end workstation. Visual display units let users consult servers and even order copies of articles. Microcomputers and high-end workstations let users download the results of their queries to their local environment and integrate them into local applications. Network computers are intermediate between dumb terminals and microcomputers.

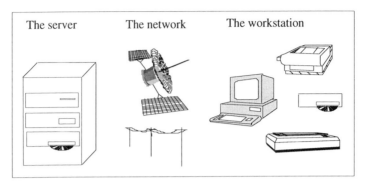

| The server | The network | The workstation |

Figure 6.1 : The technical infrastructure

Connecting to Networks

Connection may be accomplished through the telephone network, special-ized lines (e.g., ISDN, cable television lines), or over the airwaves (see Chapter 1). Network access should be immediate and transparent, whatever the destination. Ease of use has improved greatly since the beginning of the 1990s through programs such as Netscape or Internet Explorer browsers on the Internet, which provide automatic dialing, set access parameters, select servers, addressees, and communication modes (see Appendix C).

Archiving and Server Functions

Increased storage capacities let servers store ever-increasing quantities of information, even the original texts themselves, including graphics, images and sounds in the case of multimedia servers. In parallel, the multiplicity of servers has required the development of more flexible and powerful query languages, letting users ask questions in nearly natural language.

General Characteristics

Document Mediation

The objective of a documentation system is to supply to the originator of the query (e.g., physicians or a researchers) the means to access the pertinent documents for a given question (i.e., the references). The documents must have been previously indexed by specialists in the area. The indexing phase is usually performed manually, using key words defined by the authors or area specialists (documentalists) from a thesaurus of key words (Figure 6. 2). Key words are codified (see Chapter 5). They may be used alone or com-bined by logical (and, or, not), relational (greater than, equal, less than), or linkage (causes, is caused by) qualifiers which create a true artificial language. Semiautomated or automated procedures are being developed by research groups working on the analysis and comprehension of natural language to accelerate the indexing process.

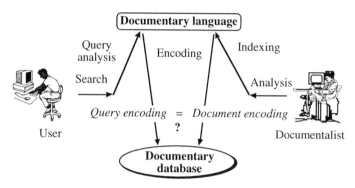

Figure 6.2 : Document mediation

When querying a document management system, the user's question undergoes an analog process that establishes a list of key words and eventual links. The success or failure of the search depends on the correlation between the two resulting encoding methods: the encoding of the query and the indexing of the document.

It is then possible to extract the bibliographic references of the selected articles (title, authors, journal, year and volume, pages, synopsis, etc.) from the document management system.

The most sophisticated systems allow the user to order copies of the articles directly, or even access the articles' full text in real time in the case of *full-text databases*.

The Quality of a Documentation Management System

The quality of a document management system may be judged not only by the pertinence and exhaustiveness of the system's replies to queries, but also by its speed and ease of use. Based on the elements illustrated in Figure 6.3, it is possible to define the following performance criteria:

The *recall rate* is defined as the number of pertinent documents (a) found out of the total number of documents in the system (a + b). For example, if 25 pertinent references exist for a given article and the system finds 20 of them, the recall rate is 20/25 or 80%. The difference between the recall rate and 100% is called the *silence*. In the preceding example, the silence equals 20%.

Normally, the recall rate and the silence are not directly measurable by the end user, who does not know the total number of pertinent documents (a) in

Documents	Found	Not found	
Pertinent	a	b	a+b
Not pertinent	c	d	c+d
	a+c	b+d	N

Figure 6.3 : Results of a document query

the system. It is possible to know the *precision* of the reply, however. Precision is defined as the number of pertinent documents a found out of the total number of documents found (a + c). In the preceding example, 20 articles were found, of which 15 are pertinent. Therefore, the precision rate is equal to 15/20 or 75%.

The difference between the precision rate and 100% is called the *noise*. It is defined as the number of nonpertinent documents found (c) out of the total number of documents found (a + c).

Besides the domain covered and the period, the major criteria for selecting a bibliographical database include the type of documents included, the frequency of updates, the depth of the information supplied, and the nature of the language used for querying the base (thesaurus or natural language).

Documentation Systems

Bibliographical Databases

Bibliographical databases have witnessed considerable growth since the mid 1960s. A bibliographical database contains the titles and references (authors, laboratory, language, etc.) of articles published in periodicals, conference notes, books, and technical reports. The rapid increase in storage capacity has enabled the addition of synopses or even the full text, as well as diagrams and figures.

Both scientific and nonscientific fields are covered. In the biomedical field, the National Library of Medicine (NLM) in Bethesda publishes over 40 databases and databanks that are accessible online. MEDLINE is certainly the most significant of these systems, and its evolution is worthy of note. MEDLINE, an abbreviation of MEDLARS (*MEDical Literature Analysis and Retrieval System*) Online, is an interactive documentary information system established by the NLM in 1971. Every year, 400,000 articles from 3,900 selected periodicals in the fields of medicine, nursing, biology, or public health are indexed with 5 to 20 terms of the MeSH (Medical Subject Headings) thesaurus (see Chapter 5). The same thesaurus is used for querying the document database. It may be accessed through a visual display screen, a microcomputer, or a workstation. There are over 9 million referenced articles dating back to 1966, 47% of which come from Europe and 5% from the Far East.

An online query of the database, using a command language, displays the number of documents in the database corresponding to the query. It may subsequently be refined, the responses viewed, and the selected references may be edited. The query may use the boolean operators (AND, OR, EXCEPT) to combine key words, authors' names, and names of periodicals. The user can receive the list of selected references by mail or photocopies of the full text (Figure 6.4).

TI: The use of multimedia in patient care.
AU: Kitanosono-T; Kurashita-Y; Honda-M; Hishida-T; Konishi-H; Mizuno-M; Anzai-M
AD: Department of Radiology, School of Medicine, Showa University, Tokyo, Japan.
SO: Comput-Methods-Programs-Biomed. 1992 May; 37(4): 259-63.
ISSN: 0169-2607
PY: 1992
LA: ENGLISH
CP: NETHERLANDS
AB: A personal computer based system was constructed to assess the use of various forms of information (multimedia) in patient record keeping. A patient's file with his records kept in a multimedia fashion was made by using the system. We describe the hardware and software construction of the system together with the Picture Archiving and Communications Systems (PACS).
MESH: Photography-; Software-;Tape-Recording; Videotape-Recording
MESH: *Medical-Records-Systems, -computerized; *Microcomputers-; *Radiology-Information-Systems
PT: JOURNAL-ARTICLE
AN: 93009664
UC: 9301

Figure 6.4 : Sample results of a MEDLINE query.
TI: document title; AU: authors; AD: address; SO: document reference; PY:
Year; LA: language; CP: country; AB: abstract; MESH: key words;
PT: type of publication; AN: access number; UC: update code

To provide easier access to the MEDLINE system, query softwares have been developed for servers, containing duplicates of the NLM files, and microcomputers (IBM compatibles or Macintosh). The PubMed software developed by the developed by the National Center for Biotechnology Information (NCBI) at the NLM is an example of this kind of software. The system that is accessible through the Internet offers menus to guide the user in formulating queries and to help save time. The search may be run using MeSH terms, more specialized terms ("children" in the MeSH hierarchy), or more general terms ("parents"). Words appearing in the titles or article summaries may also be used as access criteria. Query results may be downloaded to a microcomputer and saved for later use. Links to Web-based journals are provided for full-text retrieval.

EMBASE, the Excerpta Medica database, is a biomedical and pharmacological database which gives access to information about medical and drug-related subjects.

BIOSIS and PASCAL are other important multidisciplinary databases (Figure 6.5). They have been complemented in several areas by specialized databases, such as TOXLINE (TOXicology information onLINE) in toxicology or AIDSLINE for AIDS.

The Institute for Scientific Information (ISI) publishes citation databases, which index cited references in the footnotes or bibliographies of scientific journals (*Science Citation Index*).

The principal document or citation databases are available on CD-ROM and/or may be accessed through the Internet. Query softwares such as PubMed of Internet Grateful Med for the NLM databases allow the users to query the bases and copy the results into a word processor. In parallel, full-text databases are rapidly becoming available over networks and/or on CD-ROMs or DVD-ROMs, which include graphics and images of the principal articles.

Base	Created in	Source	Nb. of references (millions)	Scope
BIOSIS abstracts	1926	Biosis (USA)	13.5	6,000 periodicals, meetings
EMBASE	1974	Elsevier Science Publishers (Netherlands)	7.0	4,000 periodicals
MEDLINE	1966	National Library of Medicine NLM (USA)	9.0	3,900 periodicals
PASCAL	1973	CNRS (France)	9.0	9,000 periodicals, congresses, theses

Figure 6.5 : A few biomedical bibliographical databases

Medical Information and Knowledge Bases

The objective of an information base (or a knowledge base) is to supply the user with the most pertinent information possible for decision-making, such as the composition, indications, or side effects of a drug. Updates are done through successive additions, and by modifying stored data that has become obsolete. Information and knowledge bases cover all scientific and technical domains. We will only cite a few examples in medicine and biology.

In the medical area, databases may be used to perform a diagnosis or a prognosis, such as defining the optimal therapeutic strategy or toxicological surveillance. Following are several medical databases:

• In internal medicine, the ADM base, developed in Rennes, France, contains the description of signs and manifestations of 2,500 diseases [Lenoir 1981]. It is accessed by general practitioners over a Minitel terminal or the Internet.

- The BIAM (*Banque d'Information Automatisée sur les Médicaments*) contains information on nearly 3,000 chemical products and 8,000 pharmaceutical specialities. It lets users consult information on the properties of a drug or search the interactions between several drugs [Ducrot 1989]. Information may be accessed by active principle or by speciality: pharmacological properties, chemical class, action mechanisms, indications, side effects, dosages, precautions for use, manufacturer. The THERIAQUE base established by the CNIMH (*Centre National d'Information sur le Médicament Hospitalier*) in Paris has similar objectives.

- TOXNET (*TOXicology data NETwork*), published by the NLM, is a set of information and bibliographical databases on toxicology.

- PDQ (*Physician Data Query*), an information system on cancer, administered by the National Cancer Institute, has been available since 1984. It includes a file with information on cancers, their prognosis, clinical information, and treatments; a file of all ongoing therapeutic test protocols and a directory of over 10,000 physicians and more than 2,000 institutions involved in treating cancer. If no treatment is admitted for a certain stage of a cancer, the system supplies the list of research currently being evaluated. The information is validated by a group of expert oncologists. Prognostic data have been validated by over 400 specialists.

- HSTAT (*Health Services/technology Assessment Text*), distributed by the NLM, is a text database containing clinical guides.

In the field of molecular biology, access to banks of nucleic acids or proteins is indispensable for comparing nucleotide sequences or for determining the characteristics of a protein. For example, the evidence of homologous sequences among different proteins is indispensable in the study of molecular evolution and the constitution of families of proteins. The accessibility of servers on the network and the division of labor between laboratories are two steps in the enormous task of establishing the cartography of genomes of the various animal and vegetable species, including the human genome. Among the databases in this field are:

- The nucleotide base developed by the European Molecular Biology Laboratory (EMBL) in Heidelberg and the European Bioinformatics Institute in Cambridge contains over 300,000 sequences in March 1995, totalling over 260 million bases. It is updated in collaboration with the GenBank (USA) and DDBJ (Japan) bases. It doubles in size approximately every 18 months.

- EXPASY/SWISS-PROT is a database of protein sequences jointly produced by the group headed by Amos Bairoch (University of Geneva) and by the EMBL. It provides numerous annotations (e.g., a description of the function of the protein, its structure, and its variations, etc.) and links with other bases. Figure 6.6 presents a tridimensional representation of a protein.

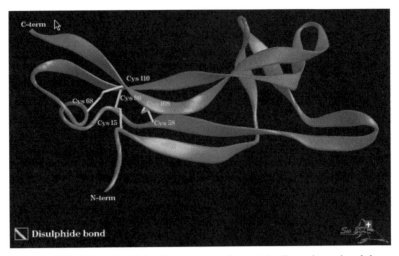

Figure 6.6 : Example of the 3D structure of a protein (Lymphotoxinealpha precursor or LT-Alph) in the ExPaSy server

- GenBank is a database of genetic sequences developed by the National Center for Biotechnology Information (NCBI), a division of the National Library of Medicine, Bethesda. GenBank contained approximately 2,162,000,000 bases in 3,044,000 sequence records in December 1998. EST sequences are partial DNA sequences that are derived from clones selected from the cDNA libraries. Figure 6.8 shows a sample EST sequence. The sequences are published in a special base, entitled dbEST.

The rapid development of multimedia technology (computers and support media) greatly facilitate the development and distribution of interactive encyclopedias on the Internet and digital optical media, such as CD-ROM or DVD-ROM. These products will provide additional information to complement the knowledge banks available over networks.

Discussion and Conclusion

The use of documentary databases and information bases was long hindered by the multiplicity of classifications and thesauri, the absence of user-friendly interfaces, and the complexity of query languages. The UMLS project [Lindberg 1993] discussed in Chapter 5 is an attempt to unify the language of medicine that will be very useful for sharing this information.

Free-form queries of databases in natural language are also an area of active research. They cover artificial intelligence methods concerning the mechanisms of comprehension, text analysis, and interpretation, as well as techniques for building voluminous dictionaries. In the future, they should provide easier access to the information sought and automatic indexing of

```
TYPE: EST
STATUS: New
CONT_NAME: Kerlavage AR
CONT_LAB: Receptor Biochemistry & Molecular Biology
EST#: EST00001
GB#: M61954
GDB#:
GDB_DSEG:
CLONE: HHC189
ATCC_INHOST: 65128
OTHER_EST: EST00093, EST000101
CITATION: Science, 252:1651 (1991)
PRIMER: M13 Forward
P_END: 5' end
DNA_TYPE: cDNA
MAP: Chromosome 1
LIBRARY: Hippocampus, Stratagene (cat. #936205)
PUBLIC: 1
PUT_ID: Actin, gamma, skeletal
COMMENT:
This is a comment about the sequence. It may contain features.
It may span several lines.
SEQUENCE:
AATCAGCCTGCAAGCAAAAGATAGGATATTCACCTACAGTGGGCACCTCCTTAAGAAGCTG
ATAGCTTGTTACACAGTAATTAGATTGAGATAATGGACACGAAACATATTCCGGGATTAAA
CATTCTTGTCAAGAAAGGGGGAGGAAGTCTGTTGTGCAAGTTTCAAAGAAAAAGGGTACCA
GCAAAAGTGATAATGATTTGAGGATTTTGTCTCTAATTGGAGGATGATTCTCATGTAAGGT
TGTTAGGAAATGGCAAAGTATTGATGATGTGTGCTATGTGATTGGTGCTAGATACTTTAAC
TGAGTATACGAGTGAAATACTTGAGACTCGTGTCACTT
||
```

Figure 6.7 : Sample protein sequence found in GenBank's EST bank

scientific texts. Thus the query function of an information bank could be transparently integrated into a larger information system such as a hospital information system or a network of physicians in a city. It would be easy to couple this with the patient's records to help documentation play a more efficient role in decision-support systems and professional training (see Chapters 12 and 13).

In parallel, the rapid development of new media for processing, storing, and consulting information should make users' jobs considerably easier and make querying document management systems and databases a routine activity.

Exercises

- *Define a document management system (reference base) and a medical information or knowledge base.*
- *Describe the minimal technical infrastructure required to access a document management system.*

- *How does one evaluate the performance of a document management system? Cite a few evaluation criteria.*
- *What is the principle for querying a document management system?*
- *Cite a few bibliographical databases.*
- *Cite a few document databases available for medicine and biology, and discuss their current and future importance.*

7

Hospital Information Systems

Introduction

A hospital information system (HIS) may be defined as a computer system designed to ease the management of all the hospital's medical and administrative information, and to improve the quality of health care. An HIS is an integrating system by vocation, and could also be called an integrated hospital information processing system (IHIPS).

The first HIS were developed in the mid-1960s in the United States and a few European countries, such as the Netherlands, Sweden or Switzerland. HIS have followed the general evolutionary trend in computing systems: the development of large central computers, the appearance of micro-computers which replaced passive terminals, the implementation of mini-computers tied together in a network, and the development of workstations and multimedia.

Although several dozen HIS are on the market, few products actually cover all the requirements of a hospital or provide adequate integration with the larger health-care networks (see Chapter 8). The diversity of the tasks to be performed, the players involved, the existing organizations, and the technical possibilities explains this situation. Nevertheless, the installation of an HIS is a necessity and may be widely supported by all the various players in a health system.

Several conditions are required to successfully implement an HIS. Some of the most important include:

- a thorough knowledge of the underlying information system of the hospital,
- a detailed analysis of the sociology of the hospital's structures and good communication, internally between the various hospital's players and externally with its environment,
- a well-adapted hardware and software strategy, and
- a good estimation of the resources necessary for its deployment and maintenance.

Analysis of the Information System

The Various Levels of the Information System

Hospitals are very complex organizations that manage considerable quantities of information. Setting up an HIS requires an in-depth analysis of the *information system of the hospital*, that is, all the interacting elements that gather, process, and supply the information necessary to the hospital's activities.

The analysis of the information system can be carried out along several different lines: What is the information system environment? What are the hospital's goals (analysis by objectives)? What is its structure and organization (structural analysis)? What functions does it offer (functional analysis)? What are the possible effects of a computer system on the hospital's organization, and how will the relationships between players be modified (behavioral analysis)?

The methodology for the analysis of a complex information system may be transposed from one country to another. This is not necessarily true for the results (all the more so for an HIS developed on the basis of diverging analyses).

The Environment of the Information System

Figure 7.1 illustrates the diversity of the players involved either directly or indirectly in the information system. These include patients, health-care personnel (physicians, nurses, paramedical personnel, pharmacists and biologists, biomedical engineers, etc.), administrative personnel, and also players outside the hospital such as organizations from government, industry, and the media.

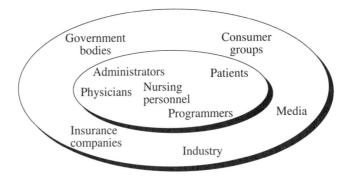

Figure 7.1 : The players involved in the hospital information system

Whatever its complexity, the hospital information system must be considered in the larger framework of the health information system in order not to underestimate the communication needs of the various subsystems (e.g., general practitioners or insurance companies). It is an essential component in the health information network and it must integrate smoothly into that network (see Chapter 8).

Figure 7.2 provides examples of the analysis levels of the information system. Most of the functions that can be computerized, such as financial planning, may be considered at several grouping levels (service, hospital, health networks, etc.).

Level	Examples of functions that may be computerized
1. Patients	Managing medical records Managing medical procedures Decision support
2. Technical-medical units	Evaluating activities Clinical research
3. Hospital	Resource planning General and cost accounting
4. Health networks	Financial planning Managing human resources
5. National	Planning for hospital expenditure Epidemiology
6. International	International comparisons

Figure 7.2 : Examples of analysis levels for information systems

HIS Objectives

Nearly everyone agrees that a hospital should primarily be considered as a set of resources employed to improve the health of the population that uses it. The same cannot be said for the secondary objectives or the detailed analysis of the institution's structure and the functions of the information system. These may vary in importance according to the various players.

Main objectives	Contributing objectives
Improve the quality of health care	Improve communications Reduce waiting times Help decision-making
Control costs	Reduce the number of days of hospitalization Reduce administrative overhead Reduce personnel expenses

Figure 7.3 : Objectives of a hospital information system (HIS)

Most players agree that the HIS is a means to improve health care while providing a more rational management of medical activities. Insurance companies may hope that the HIS will provide a better understanding of the hospital's activities and the health needs of the population. They hope to include mobile health care and care at home in a more rational system for controlling costs (Figure 7.3). If security and respect for individual rights can be guaranteed (see Chapters 8 and 15), opening an HIS to the outside may be a way to decompartmentalize medicine in and outside the hospital and to bring medicine closer to the patient.

Structural Analysis

The structural analysis must include a detailed analysis of the organization, material and human resources. In France, the material structure and the hierarchical human resources (services) are interdependent. In North America, on other hand, the material resources (beds, ancillary departments) are shared between the various human resources (departments) (Figure 7.4).

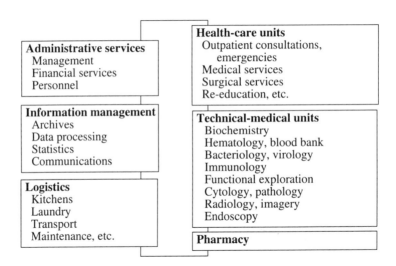

Figure 7.4 : Hospital organization

In principle, a medical-technical service, unlike a traditional health-care unit, is not responsible for following patients. In practice, the last ten years experience shows that the distinction between a medical-technical service and a clinical service is not always so clear-cut. A laboratory may handle certain categories of patients (e.g., hemophiliacs or patients taking anticoagulants for a hematology service). Inversely, a clinical service may develop an exploratory activity for the rest of the hospital or for outside structures (e.g., echocardiography, endoscopy, etc.).

When analyzing an information system, every structure, medical or medical-technical, becomes a resource available to the other structures or to the outside, performing medical acts, producing information, or consuming other resources.

Functional Analysis

Functional analysis helps to define a system's various functions (medical diagnostic or therapeutic activities, managing resources, etc.). It defines the WHAT of the information system.

The existence of the necessary structures is a prerequisite for effective performance of a function (the HOW). A good analysis of the objectives and functions often raises questions about the existing organization. In a complex system, some structures evolve for their own needs while moving away from their objectives, or they evolve without any direct link to the total system's objectives. Sometimes, on the contrary, indispensable structures are set up belatedly (e.g., due to inadequacy of the information management system).

Any division of the hospital's information system into subsystems is arbitrary. We can distinguish three major approaches:

- The first and most widely used method bases subsystems on hospital structures. It differentiates the medico-administrative information subsystem from the health-care subsystem or the ancillary services subsystem (biology, radiology, etc.). This method is usually appreciated by the players because it naturally adapts itself to the hospital's organization. It has led to the development of departmental systems. It promotes the idea of a health-care team (physicians, nurses, and paramedical personnel) and network dynamics within the hospital. It does have certain disadvantages, however. It tends to split the patient information system among the different subsystems. It may lead to the development of redundant or even incoherent applications (e.g., different functions for managing requests for examinations, and applications for managing health-care units or ancillary departments).

- The second approach reflects the functions of the players in the information system. It helps identify the needs of the various categories of hospital personnel. This method deals with administrative, medical, nursing, and other information subsystems. If precautions are not taken when developing computer applications, this method may lead to redundant functions and sometimes to contradictions that hinder optimal patient care (e.g., isolating the medical records from the nursing records).

- The third approach differentiates the *patient information subsystem* (anything that concerns the patient and that may be stored in the patient's record) from the other subsystems. Figure 7.5 illustrates this approach. The functions in the right-hand column are directly related to the patients' medical care, while the left-hand column concerns functions related to the hospital and its structures. This method emphasizes the notion of the unique patient record, which acts as the basis for administrative, medical or nursing information, and for decision-making (see Chapter 9). It also has the advantage of centering the analysis on the hospital's main objective, improving the health of its patients and optimizing their care. It is the root of hospital information systems built around patient records.

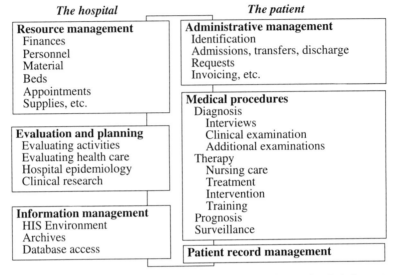

Figure 7.5 : Functional analysis: the individualization of the patient's information subsystem

The Components of an HIS

We will present brief summaries of the traditional components of an HIS.

Administration

This includes the medico-administrative patient management subsystems, general and cost accounting, human resource management, inventory control, and purchasing (Figure 7.6).

Health-Care Units

These units group functions related to patient health care and medical activities in general (Figure 7.7). They are therefore very complex and difficult to model. We may divide these units into three sub-systems:

- the subsystem that carries out actions (requesting examinations, returning results);
- the subsystem that creates the permanent patient record; and
- the subsystem that controls and pilots these activities.

- **Medico-administrative patient management**
  - Identification
  - Preadmission, admission, discharge, transfers
  - Invoicing, links with insurance companies
- **Financial management**
  - General and cost accounting
  - Administrative controls
- **Inventory management**
  - Purchasing
  - Planning
- **Hospital activities management**
  - Resource management (beds, appointments)
  - Activity/statistical reports (range of cases)
  - Resource planning and optimization
- **Personnel management**

Figure 7.6 : The administrative subsystem

Communication functions are very important. Part of their complexity is related to the need to tie together information concerning health-care procedures performed both inside and outside the hospital in order to avoid redundant examinations and to guarantee coherent care.

- **Managing patient data**
  - Observations, interviews, examinations, diagnostic and prognostic decisions, etc.)
  - Procedure management (prescriptions and procedures)
  - Reporting (reports, file summaries, charts)
- **Health care management**
  - Logistics
  - Administration and accounting
  - Statistics on activities
- **Communications**
  - Internal and external health care units
  - Outside the hospital
- **Training and research**
  - Access to knowledge, protocols
  - Querying data banks

Figure 7.7 : The health-care unit subsystem

Ancillary Departments

This label covers all the activities of the biology laboratories, functional exploration services, and imaging services. Figure 7.8 displays the functions managed by these units.

- **Examinations**
  - Recording requests
  - Printing documents -> technical stations
  - Data acquisition
    Manual
    Connection to analyzers
  - Validation
  - Printing and distribution
  - Archiving
- **Laboratory management**
  - Administration and accounting
  - Quality control
  - Statistics on activities

Figure 7.8 : The biological information system

Strategies and Technical Solutions

The Vertical Approach: Centralized HIS

The first systems, implemented during the 1970s, used this design [Ball 1980]. These systems are usually characterized by a centralized architecture, supplied by a single manufacturer, made up of a central computer and peripherals arranged in a star-shaped network (Figure 7.9). They attempt to integrate all hospital functions in a single hardware and software architecture.

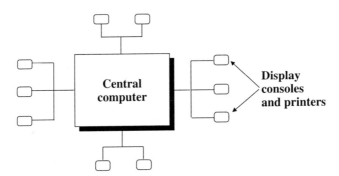

Figure 7.9 : HIS architecture in star configuration

Peripherals like the IBM PC are a natural evolution of this architecture. This hardware architecture has its software equivalent: hierarchical database management systems (DMBS) like IBM's *DL1* used in the Patient Care System (PCS). A few simple principles dominate this architecture. Information is only entered once, is stored in a single place in the central database (the nonredundancy principle), and is accessible from any place in the network (the shared data principle). Data protection is simplified. Complementary units, such as minicomputers for managing laboratories, may be connected in a star to the central machine.

TDS was one of the first demonstrative installations of this type. It was put in service in the early 1970s in the El Camino Hospital in California, and then spread to over a hundred hospitals in North America and Europe. In this system, terminals or PCs are used to enter the information required for medico-administrative management and patient surveillance. When a physician prescribes an urgent biological examination, a test order form is automatically printed on the printer attached to the terminal of the nurse in charge of the patient, as well as the labels to identify the samples. The laboratory is simultaneously alerted of the arrival of the sample. Once the sample has been tested and validated, the results are directly transmitted to the patient's biological record without human intervention. The physician can query the system at any time to know the results. The HIS system offers real-time access to several data banks (e.g., medications, guide for prescribing antibiotics, guides for indicating and interpreting complementary examinations, etc.). The records for nursing care are very complete and well-integrated in the HIS.

The HELP system, developed at the University of Utah in Salt Lake City and commercialized by the 3M Company, is organized around an intelligent dictionary. It was the first system to offer alarm and protocol management directly controlled by the data (see Chapter 12) [Pryor 1987].

The vertical, centralized approach, has a number of advantages:

• The HIS is truly integrated and centered on unique patient records.

• It facilitates the installation and maintenance of application modules.

• It satisfies the administrators, who see this as a simple method for controlling their institution; the data processing staff, who see it as a means of controlling larger and larger computers; and the manufacturers, who try to ensure their customers' loyalty. It is not easy to change a centralized architecture based on a preferred vendor with specific software from that vendor. These represent considerable investments for equipping a computing center, as does the training of the development teams and maintenance.

This approach is usually included in proposals for "turnkey" systems.

A centralized architecture does have a number of disadvantages, however:

• It makes the institution highly dependent on a single manufacturer, or on an HIS vendor/manufacturer pair.

• The computing installation cannot develop progressively but only in leaps, when the central computer is updated or changed.

• Users' specific needs are only partially satisfied.

• The centralized nature of the single database requires exaggerated standardization which may in itself hinder any development initiatives.

The Horizontal Approach: Departmental Systems

The horizontal approach involves the purchase of specialized applications for the various structures in the hospital. The medico-technical units, in particular the biochemical and hematology laboratories, were the first to follow the administrative services and benefit from this departmental approach. Computerizing the health-care units is more complex. The requirements of the medical corps vary, and it is difficult to establish a "body of information" acceptable to the rather large user community.

This approach has several advantages:

- It provides products better adapted to user requirements, as users may choose from the large number of products on the market. It is also possible for each service to use the best hardware–software combination.
- Progressive investment is made possible through the successive acquisition of different applications and, for an institution that groups several hospitals, by economies of scale for distributing a single product across several sites.
- Data can be grouped together, and multicentric clinical research programs can be established (in the case of several services in the same speciality).

These advantages explain the horizontal approach's varying levels of success in several multihospital institutions, where a return on investment can be expected from the deployment in units sharing the medical domain, and especially in university teaching hospitals, where the flexibility of the approach facilitates clinical research.

The horizontal approach also has its drawbacks. The choice of the most appropriate system at a given time for a given discipline may lead to an information system that resembles the Tower of Babel and to the installation of incompatible hardware or software architectures. The cost of integrating heterogeneous applications may significantly overrun the operational cost of a vertical system.

The Distributed Approach: Distributed and Open Systems

The mixed approach attempts to combine the advantages (and hopefully not the disadvantages) of the vertical and horizontal approaches. Applications, defined in terms of the major functions of the HIS, are distributed over several processors in a distributed, "open" architecture operating in *client-server* mode (Figure 7.10) [Scherrer 1990, Van de Velde 1992]. The location of functional HIS modules is transparent to the user (*distributed architecture*). This may include patient identity servers, laboratory results, clinical data (e.g., hospitalization reports and diagnostic encoding), or images servers (see Chapter 11). The functional components are selected from existing elements, which usually must be adapted, or from off-the-shelf products in order to take advantage of the best hardware–software combination, as in the departmental approach. In principle, changing a module does not require a change in the HIS's general architecture.

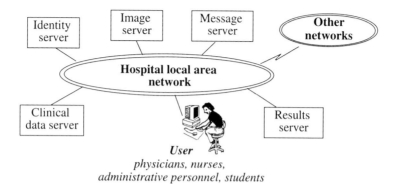

Figure 7.10 : Example of a server-based HIS architecture

The complexity of the actual implementation for this approach nevertheless requires the choice of an appropriate hardware, software, and network architecture. The choice of operating systems, networking standards, and man–machine interfaces, which should remain independent of a given manufacturer, is particularly important.

The development of multimedia workstations is an important component of this type of approach, both for facilitating the visualization (e.g., through Web browsers) and management of complex medical objects and for hiding the complexity of the underlying information system (see Figure 7.11) [Hammond 1990, Safran 1994, Van Mulligen 1995].

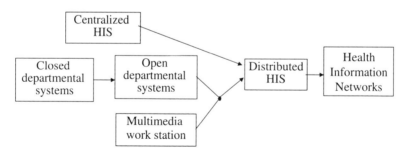

Figure 7.11 : Evolution of HIS architectures

Distributing functions across several servers requires a certain redundancy of information that must be handled by the selected database management system. Applications must be able to communicate between themselves by messages whose contents must have been previously standardized (see Chapter 1). New software products, often named under the generic term of *middleware* need to be developed to guaranty the syntactic and semantic interoperability of the system components.

All these constraints explain why no perfectly operational distributed information system exists today.

Required Resources

Allocating Resources and Estimating Costs

Estimating the costs of installing and operating an HIS and the evolution of those costs is a difficult task. Even hospitals that make the most extensive use of information technology are still in a phase of rapid growth of their information systems. The number of information workstations, the volume of communications with the appearance of image transfers, and the storage capacities due to the arrival of digital optical media, are all growing rapidly. The share of the average operating budget dedicated to computing is on the order of 1% to 1.5% for French hospitals, far lower than the budgets in the United States (in the neighborhood of 2% to 3%) [Dorenfest 1995].

Company	Administrative management \# sites and %	Health-care management \# sites and %
HBOC (HBO and PCS)	647 (22.0%)	498 (21.9%)
SMS	632 (21.5%)	482 (21.1%)
First Data	281 (9.6%)	213 (9.3%)
Meditech	251 (8.5%)	232 (10.2%)
Alltel (Systematics/TDS)	68 (2.3%)	127 (5.6%)
Management Systems Associates	47 (1.6%)	31 (1.4%)
Number of hospitals having a system	2,938 (100%)	2,279 (100%)

Figure 7.12 : Hospital information systems market in the USA. 2,938 hospitals with more than 100 beds in 1994. (Adapted from [Dorenfest 1995])

Figure 7.12 provides a glimpse of the HIS in the 2,938 American hospitals with over 100 beds [Dorenfest 1995]. 100% of these hospitals have an administrative management system and 77.6% have a health-care management system. Health-care management systems essentially cover the management of care (e.g., ordering acts, displaying results, and producing inpatient summary records) and the control of these activities (e.g., through case mix). Computerized patient records are more limited.

Human Resources

Managing human resources is one of the keys to success for an HIS. One must ensure the smooth integration of administrative, hospital, and university staff, provide the human resources required for the development and correct operation of the HIS, and prepare all personnel for its use.

Several hospitals support a dual computing system where administrative computing (e.g., invoicing patients for hospitalization, payroll, economic management) is separated from medical computing. The analysis of the hospital's information system shows that maintaining this duality is contrary to the very objectives of an HIS. A piece of information, such as the age of a patient, can be administrative or medical according to how it is used. The success of certain American experiments, such as those at Harvard (Beth Israel) and the LDS Hospital in Salt Lake City, or European efforts such as at the Cantonal University Hospital in Geneva (HCUG) with the Diogène system or the AZ-VUB in Brussels, may be partly due to the constantly reinforced desire to regroup administrative, hospital, and university human resources around common goals. The various implementation phases of an HIS must also be supported by the research teams, particularly in university hospitals.

Discussion and Conclusion

A certain number of tools, either currently available or under development in research laboratories, should provide considerable improvements over the coming years. None of them today is considered as the ultimate answer, given the significant difference between the possibilities of these tools and the real needs of the medical community. The terminals still used in certain hospital information systems (24 lines, 80 columns per line) do not permit a satisfactory dialogue with the computer. The use of microcomputers as access terminals to an HIS provides additional but nonetheless insufficient comfort. The development of low-cost medical workstations with sophisticated graphics and networking capabilities is a challenge of the next decade.

Decision-support techniques and the implementation of knowledge base systems have developed in parallel with database management systems. They have been demonstrated to facilitate medical decision-making and improve the quality of care. Fifteen years after testing the first prototypes, the number of operational systems remains small, and the investments required to update knowledge bases are considerable.

The best HIS cannot function without the active participation of all personnel concerned. Their participation must start in the analysis phase, or individuals may refuse to participate at a later stage. It implies adequate training of all personnel (i.e., medical, nursing, and administrative). This training must go beyond an introduction to personal productivity software, electronic mail, or practical training on an operational HIS. It must also analyze the organizational consequences of the strategic choices decided in common. The HIS can create a human network that is just as important as the electronic communication network, if not more so.

Exercises

- *Define the objectives and the principal functions of a hospital information system.*
- *List the advantages that a hospital information system can provide.*
- *How is the information concerning biological and radiological examinations circulated within the hospital? What steps will most benefit from automation or computerization?*
- *List the major functions of a health-care unit management system.*
- *Know the advantages and disadvantages of centralized, departmentalized, and distributed hospital information systems.*
- *What are the principal problems involved with implementing a hospital information system?*

8

Health-Care Networks

Introduction

Developed countries face major changes in health care. The exponential growth of new techniques for medical investigation and treatment contribute to this evolution, as does the rapid increase in the number of medical personnel and the reorganization of the health-care providers in an attempt to manage the cost and quality of health care.

These changes lead to increasingly complex systems for health care and for distributing information. Medical data concerning an individual may be produced at the hospital or the patient's home, in the doctor's office or at the workplace. The traditional one-to-one relationship that existed previously between patient and physician has changed into a one-to-many relationship. This type of networked relationship is becoming the norm between health-care professionals and the health insurance organizations. It requires a strategy for sharing and communicating information that must accommodate three often contradictory elements:

- *The quality of health care.* Improving the quality of care requires good communication among health-care personnel and easily accessible, reliable, and integrated information, including linkage of patient-related information. The hospital is only one of the links in the health-care chain. The search for quality must be viewed in a more global fashion, up the entire length of the chain. It requires a detailed analysis of the activity of the various links in the chain, their coherence, and their complementarity (see Chapter 14).

- *Training and research.* Information systems that help identify and follow patients belonging to different health-care structures are required to improve knowledge, to evaluate the results of procedures, and to implement global training. Chronic diseases, the importance of establishing reliable registers (e.g., for cancers), and warning systems (e.g., for transmissible diseases) are particularly important examples of this requirement.

- *Health finances and organization.* Cost control requires a reorganization of health-care providers and better control of distribution. To simplify, three sectors may be considered: inpatient care, outpatient care, and home care and patient self-care (Figure 8.1). Reductions in health-care expenses are mainly obtained by controlling hospital expenses (section 3 in Figure 8.1) where most of the expensive experts and procedures are located. But this reduction may transfer the expenses to out-patient care (section 2 in Figure 8.1) and have negative effects on the quality of care. Patients must also be prepared to participate more actively in the health-care process, and eventually to manage without the physician's direct intervention (i.e., avoid sections 2 and 3 in Figure 8.1) whenever that is not prejudicial to their health.

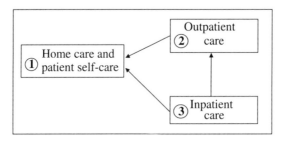

Figure 8.1 : Strategies for reducing the cost of health care

The Health System

Health-Care Coverage

The organization of the health-care system varies enormously from country to country. The differences may concern the principal subsystems that make up the health-care network, patient demand, the social coverage system, and the control and/or regulation mechanisms.

In the French health-care system, approximately 8.5% of the gross domestic product (GDP) was dedicated to health expenses in 1987, while in 1994 the total was 9.7%. This represents $2,600 annually per capita (Figure 8.2). Nearly all patients (99%) have health-care coverage, but the reimbursement rate has gradually diminished and is now around 70%. Approximately 75% of reimbursements are covered by Social Security, 5% by mutual insurance companies, and 20% by private insurance. In 1994, there were approximately 1,000 public hospitals representing 360,000 beds and 2,400 private hospitals and clinics with 195,000 beds. Patients in France are free to choose their health-care facility.

In the United States, 10.8 percent of the GDP was spent on health care in 1987 and nearly 15% in 1995, representing approximately $3,000 annually per capita, with significant regional variation. In 1990, 65% of these costs were covered by private financing and 35% by public spending. Medicare and Medicaid, the two large public health insurance systems, are managed by the Health Care Financing Administration (HCFA).

	USA	France†
Total population (millions)	263	58
Gross domestic product (billions of US dollars)	5400	1400
Health care spending (billions of US dollars)	800	140
Percentage of the population without health coverage	15%	1%
Number of hospitals	6,600	3,400
Number of hospital beds/1000 inhabitants	4.7	9.7
Number of employees per bed (in 1990)	3.4	1.1
Total number of physicians (thousands)	700	190
Number of inhabitants per physician	375	305
Generalists (%)	20%	30%
Estimated number of physicians in 2010 (thousands)	825	205

† Calculations are based on 1 US dollar = 5.5 FF

Figure 8.2 : Comparison of two health-care systems (based on 1994 estimates)

The budget for *Medicare,* the system created in the United States in 1965 under the Johnson administration for citizens over 65 years of age, has grown continuously. In 1994, it totalled $114 billion, representing 17% of health-care expenses. Since 1983, this system reimburses for hospitalizations on a fixed-rate basis, determined by a classification in one of the *diagnostic related groups* (DRGs) (see Chapter 14). *Medicaid*, the second system, was also established in 1965. It provides coverage for 25 million Americans living in poverty (those with income between $200 and $1,000 per month, depending on the state), and its budget totalled $150 billion in 1994. Approximately 35 million Americans (15% of the population) living just above the poverty level have no health-care coverage and can only be treated in emergencies. Due to lack of "portability" of Americans' health insurance, citizens lose their existing coverage when they change employers or become unemployed. Recently introduced legislation may broaden this coverage in the future.

Medical Demographics

The total number of physicians in France quadrupled between 1950 and 1990. In 1995, the total was near 190,000, which represents one physician for every 305 inhabitants, with strong regional differences (from 1 to 3). In 1988, 55% were independents, and 30% mainly salaried employees. 70% of physicians are specialists, a situation similar to most other European countries except for Great Britain, where the percentage does not exceed 25%. The great majority of physicians work for fees based on agreements established between medical syndicates and Social Security. In Sector 1, which includes three quarters of the independents, fees are determined by the convention; social charges for the physician are low, and patients are reimbursed for approximately 70% of the cost of the visit. Physicians in Sector 2 are allowed to exceed the fixed rates, but their social charges are higher; patient reimbursements are made on the same basis as for Sector 1. A very small number of physicians operate outside the convention. They are free to set their fees, but the Social Security reimbursements are minimal. Physicians are increasingly creating group offices and networks including both generalists and specialists (Figure 8.3).

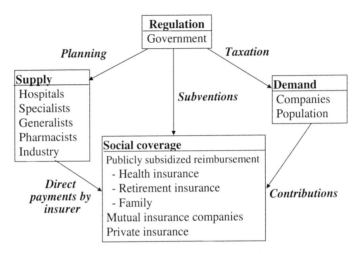

Figure 8.3 : The French health-care system

In the United States, the total number of physicians tripled between 1950 and 1990, reaching approximately 700,000 in 1995, with a very high percentage of specialists (75%). The excess number of physicians could be greater than 150,000 in the year 2000, especially for specialists. *Health Maintenance Organizations* (HMOs), created in 1973 under the Nixon administration, are a primary example of a health-care network where an insurance group, usually private, creates contracts with individual physicians and/or groups of private physicians and hospitals to provide global health care (both outpatient care and hospitalization, prevention, physical therapy, etc.). In this system, patient fees are annual and individual, per *capita*. Physicians must respect health protocols that attempt to limit expenses (known as *managed care*) with or without bonuses for efficiency. In 1993, over 75% of physicians worked for one or several HMOs. The number of patients enrolled in HMOs has grown from 6 million in 1976 to nearly 70 million in 1995. In this highly competitive environment, teaching hospitals are in trouble because their hospitalization costs are higher than those of general hospitals. They often join forces in an attempt to improve productivity but at the expense of teaching and research functions. Many establish contracts with groups of physicians, and in some cases create their own structures similar to HMOs.

Health-Care Networks and Health Information Systems

The Components of a Health-Care Network

A health-care network may be viewed as a group of players and resources dedicated to providing quality health care (Figure 8.4). The resources (hospitals, outpatient care, insurance companies, etc.) are heterogeneous and interdependent [Launois 1986]. Organizing these resources into coordinated care structures is now viewed as necessary to guarantee quality and efficiency. In the United States, the term CHIN (for *community health information network*) is normally used to designate the computer infrastructure required for proper operation of a health-care network.

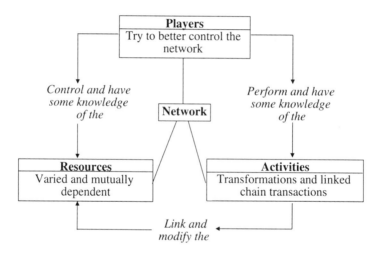

Figure 8.4 : The players-activities-resources triad (adapted from [Hakansson 1989])

Figure 8.5 illustrates the three main components in a health-care network and their relationship:

- *The communication and storage system* (level 1 of Figure 8.5). The health-care network is based on a technological infrastructure including a communications network, resources for storing and processing information (application servers), and network access points (professional workstations). Chapter 1 describes the operation of these elements.

- *The system to provide health care* (level 2 of Figure 8.5). This system is centered around the patient. It involves the intervention of the various categories of health-care professionals. It must provide indicators required for the medical and economic management of the system. The system must be implemented in a way that is satisfactory to both the legal system and professional ethics.

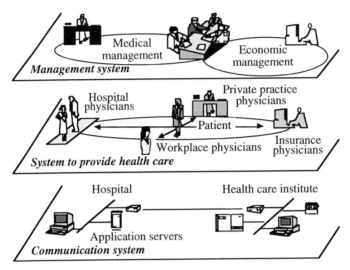

Figure 8.5 : Functional and technical architecture of a health-care network

- *The management system* (level 3 of Figure 8.5). It requires a vision of the future of the network that may be applied to the activity and quality indicators. This system particularly concerns medical, administrative, or political decision-makers. Public or private organizations may control the finances.

Telemedicine Tools in Health-Care Networks

In a health-care network, the health-care enterprise becomes a *virtual enterprise*, defined at any given time by a set of players and resources in dynamic interaction, linked by the network. In this framework, the need to share medical knowledge and patient data is obvious. Three types of computer applications meet these requirements, normally grouped under the name of telemedicine:

- *Teleconsultations* (or remote consultations) attempt to reduce the distance between the patient, the physician, and the specialist. They require a high level of interaction between the person requesting information (patient, generalist, or health-care personnel) and the person being consulted (health-care personnel, generalist, or specialist). They mainly use messaging and interactive video techniques. *Tele-expertise* (remote consultation with an expert) is particularly used to interpret X-ray images (*teleradiology*) or pathological images (*telepathology*). *Tele-education* concerns patient education or professional medical or paramedical training.

- *Telesurveillance* (or remote surveillance) remotely collects surveillance parameters and can even remotely control objects. It can facilitate home surveillance for chronically ill patients, offering an alternative to hospitalization. Specialities such as nephrology, for home dialysis, and pulmonary medicine, for management of respiratory deficiencies, are particularly suited to these techniques.
- *Groupware (*or collaborative work tools) require interactive video functions, messaging tools and reading and updating full patient records.

Data Access and Communications

Workstations and the Communication Environment

Accessing the health-care network, either from a medical office or a patient's home, requires a microcomputer or a workstation, along with communication tools to connect to the telephone network (or using radio waves) to access the various data servers and to send and receive messages. This hardware may also include input-output peripherals (e.g., a video camera for telemedicine, a printer for printing reports). Although the cost of the hardware has dropped dramatically over the past few years, the cost of software increases constantly, and today exceeds hardware costs.

The availability of integrated services digital network (ISDN) and high-speed networks enables the transmission and reception of digitized images. Image compression techniques and the development of high-speed networks (asynchronous transfer mode or ATM) make possible the transmission of video sequences, and videoconferences may be used for group discussions for clinical cases or for training sessions.

The standardization of message formats and the development of standards for exchanging data (*Electronic Data Interchange* or EDI) are prerequisites for reducing the administrative costs related to network management. This concerns the exchange of both medical messages and administrative forms.

Smart Cards

The use of *smart cards*, based on the model of banking cards with a built-in microprocessor, has several possible applications in health-care networks. For the health professional, it may serve as an instrument for identification and authentication, a *professional health card* (PHC)*,* that authorizes access to medical computer files in hospitals or professional data servers. For the patient, it may serve as a method of payment for medical fees or medications and as a medium for storing critical information such as blood type or allergies. In Germany, a standardized social security card was successfully made available for every patient in 1994.

Extensive use of smart cards as a method of payment requires a major reorganization of the health information system and the reimbursement system in particular. It is easy to imagine the impact such a system could have on improving the transparency of medical activities and eliminating the transcription of redundant information such as prescriptions, Social Security forms, etc.

The use of smart cards as portable storage devices for medical records poses the problem of defining standards for card contents and for encoding information, as well as the problem of the availability of readers across the entire health-care network.

The Information System for Generalists

The Key Role of the Generalist in the Health-Care Network

Whatever the health-care system, the generalist is at the heart of the network. He or she must interact with the hospital system, the test laboratories, the paramedical environment (dentists, private nurses, physical therapists, etc.), the pharmaceutical sector, and insurance organizations. As the front-line physician, the generalist is also responsible for all of a patient's problems and for ongoing care. In fact, the generalist fulfills important and complementary functions:

- *diagnostic and evaluation functions:*

  - making diagnoses or selecting the pathological area to help orient the patient in the health system;

  - evaluating the severity of the case;

  - acting as a *gatekeeper*, if necessary calling upon the secondary health-care system (specialists from public or private hospitals, or independents);

- *patient surveillance functions:*

  - supervising pregnancies;

  - treating chronically ill patients, whose numbers will only increase with the advancing age of the general population;

- *screening, prevention, and education functions* such as establishing a vaccination schedule, managing risk factors, and screening for certain types of cancer;

- *medical-legal functions* such as making mandatory declarations of certain pathologies, preparing medical-legal certificates (workplace accidents, pregnancies, aptitude for sports, death certificates, etc.);

- eventually *evaluation and research functions:*

  - gathering epidemiological information for research or health organizations (e.g., regional health observatories);

- participating in clinical research such as evaluating diagnostic or therapeutic procedures in collaboration with the public or private sector (e.g., pharmaceutical laboratories);

- pharmaceutical supervision;

- evaluating medical practices (see Chapter 14).

Computerizing the Doctor's Office

Administrative and Financial Management

This is the area that receives the most attention from software designers and users. Most of the management functions for medical offices can be computerized:

- recording activities;
- managing appointments, especially for group offices and specialists' appointments that may require further treatment;
- maintaining registries and mandatory records (income, expenses, etc.);
- managing deferred payments (public and private insurance);
- tax declarations.

Office Automation

These software products can directly assist with repetitive tasks such as writing certificates, letters (e.g., to other physicians, recall letters, etc.), prescriptions, or simple protocols (health and dietary recommendations, possible side-effects for medications, conditions for performing further examinations, etc.).

Managing Patient Records

Computerizing patient records for generalists raises all the problems of transferring any medical record system to a computer (see Chapter 9). Additional problems are caused by the brevity of consultations, especially for family practice, the material difficulties of data entry (in particular when visiting patients at home), and the absence of a standard nomenclature of medical terms adapted to medical practice outside hospitals that is accepted nationally and internationally.

The limited amount of time that can be spent entering information leads either to the selection of a limited amount of coded information or to entering in plain text, which makes later use difficult.

Although the International Classification of Diseases has been adapted to encoding hospitalizations (ICD9-CM), it is poorly suited to encoding the activities of a generalist, where medical symptomatology plays an important role. A number of codification systems have been proposed, such as the International Classification of Health Process in Primary Care (ICPC-2) established by the *World Organization of National Colleges and Academies* (WONCA) [WONCA 1998] or the Read codes (or Clinical Terms) version 3 [NHS 1995], but none have achieved international acceptance.

Medical Decision-Support Systems

Medical decision-support systems require an initial search for standardized information on the patient, which in turn requires the availability of the physician and powerful yet easy-to-use software. The most significant experiments have involved:

- preparing diagnoses, such as the QMR program for internal medicine (see Chapter 12);
- assistance in prescribing medication (e.g., a search for a contra-indications or interactions);
- access to factual knowledge (i.e., how to react to a medical problem, therapeutic protocols, coupling with a bibliographical system, etc.).

Communication with the Outside World

Ideally, communications functions concern:

- access to the hospital sector to recover complete or partial medical records;
- access to public or private laboratory data for consulting and/or recovering the results of additional examinations;
- access to bibliographical databases or information databases (see Chapter 6);
- exchanging professional information with colleagues, insurance organizations, research or epidemiological centers, or patients;
- participation in epidemiological studies (e.g., watchdog physicians), or evaluation studies requiring the collaboration of several physicians [Valleron 1993].

Permanent Education

This is a potentially important area given the modern multimedia technologies available in microcomputer systems (see Chapters 1 and 13). Its use depends on the optional or mandatory nature of the training and the existence of a system for renewing accreditations.

The Patient's Information System

The patient's information system should be viewed from two perspectives:

- the more passive view, that of home care, which may be considered either as an extension or an alternative to inpatient or outpatient healthcare.

- the more active view, where patients become involved in their own health care. This self-care system starts with training and leads to therapeutic adaptation or even autodiagnosis and medication.

Integrating the patient into the health-care network obviously creates the problem of justifying the purchase of a home computer. In France, the availability of Videotex terminals (over 7 million Minitel terminals were in place in 1995) has led to the creation of a communication culture. The availability of networks of networks such as the Internet, falling cost of home computers or low cost new devices such as network computers and television computers points towards a second generation of applications in patients' homes. The following examples are representative of this trend.

Active Participation in Health Care

- Consulting and updating medical records: patients measure and enter medical data such as weight, blood pressure, or glycemia for hypertensive or diabetic patients [Billault 1995].
- Therapeutic adjustments, or even self-medication, within the framework of protocols defined in agreement with health-care professionals (e.g., diabetics or patients with kidney failure).

Training at Home

- Access to databases and knowledge bases available over the Internet.
- Active participation in training programs.

Electronic Messaging

- The use of electronic messaging between the patient and health-care professionals.
- The establishment of electronic forums between patients on specific themes such as AIDS, Alzheimer's disease, or genetic diseases.

Discussion and Conclusion

The uncontrolled growth of medical expenses, without parallel increases in quality of care or in the health of the general population, requires major reforms of health-care systems. These reforms, which involve the participation of all the players, must avoid two pitfalls:

- ultraliberalism, which may lead to several different quality levels of medicine and may prevent redistribution of productivity gains in a "profit-oriented business" logic. This may lead to the exclusion of a significant proportion of the population from the protection system, and finally to a social fracture.

- excessive state control, which may lead to rationed, low-quality health care for all.

In any case, the creation of integrated health-care networks seems to be the only solution for coordinating the activities of the various sectors of the health industry (inpatient, outpatient and home care, social protection system, etc.). The community health information networks represent the computing infrastructure. Their implementation has been made possible through the development of communication networks. When a society spends more than $3,000 per capita each year on health, the purchase of a microcomputer to connect the players to the network no longer appears as a major economic obstacle, especially for the targeted players (e.g., health-care professionals, high-risk patients).

Although today's computer technology is capable of integrating both the generalist and the patient in a network connecting all the players in the health-care system, several factors continue to hinder the development of these networks. Users must carefully consider the costs of communication and access to servers, must evaluate the time required for formulating questions or messages, and in general, must consider the amount of training required to use communication software and servers. Data exchange standards are under development. Real problems concerning individual privacy and guarantees of patient freedoms have arisen and require solutions (see Chapter 15). As in other sectors, technology precedes the general establishment of a medical culture that integrates the networked processing of information and the ethics for managing that information.

Exercises

- *Define a health-care network.*
- *Cite a few arguments that encourage the development of health-care networks.*
- *Cite a few applications for telemedicine in a health-care network.*
- *Define the information system for a physician working outside the hospital. What is the role of the generalist in a health-care network?*
- *List the principal functions in a doctor's office that may be computerized.*
- *Discuss the problems presented by the distance of doctors' offices from health centers and large ancillary departments and the solutions offered by computers and telecommunications.*
- *What are the factors that may discourage physicians from integrating computers into their offices?*
- *Discuss the role that patients can play in the development of health-care networks.*

9

Managing Patient Records

Introduction

Patient records are the repository where all the information required for patient care and surveillance is stored (Figure 9.1). As a tool for *memorization*, records are a central element in health care, and their development follows the more general evolution of the practice of medicine. The information they store is increasingly complex, reflecting the appearance of new methods of investigation, in particular signal analysis, imaging and molecular medicine (see Chapters 10 and 11). Records are physically distributed (e.g., among hospitals, general practitioners, or insurance organizations) and shared among health professionals. They are a necessary a tool for *communication*.

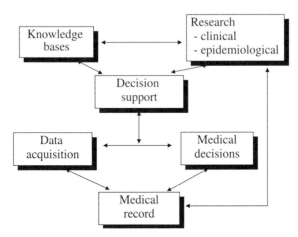

Figure 9.1 : The key position of patient records

When used individually, they directly take part in *decision-making*. Used collectively, they represent the experience of the health-care teams and may be used as tools for *evaluation*, *research,* or *planning*.

Given the pace of technological change, computerizing patient records remains a difficult undertaking but not an impossible one. It may maximize the functionality of traditional records but initially requires redoubled efforts. On the one hand, the information system must be analyzed and the needs of various user categories must be carefully evaluated. On the other hand, medical data and knowledge must be standardized and structured.

Different Views of Patient Records

All those concerned in the health system are closely involved with patient records, but the data used reflects a number of different situations and partial views of the records (Figures 9.2 and 9.3).

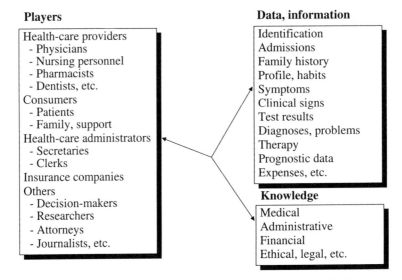

Figure 9.2 : Categories of players, information, and knowledge

The various health personnel — care providers — are directly involved. They participate daily in updating the patient's record and use it directly to make medical decisions.

Patients, of course, are those most directly concerned by the existence of high-quality records, to ensure the transmission of information required for the continuity of their care. Records help guarantee the quality of care and may serve as educational documents. For certain types of data, patients may directly take part in updating the information (see Chapter 8).

Administrators and social organizations are more concerned with the social and economic elements, as well as the evaluation of the quality or the productivity of the health-care system. Public health specialists see the patient record as a clinical or epidemiological research tool (in case studies, for example).

Each category of player, with its own view of the patient record, tends to favor certain functions of a computerized record. We may therefore talk about the medical record, the nursing record, or the administrative record (Figure 9.3). It should be noted that the same information (age or sex, for example) may be of a medical, nursing, or administrative nature according to how it is used, and that it is probably in the patient's best interest to provide a single integrated view of the patient record.

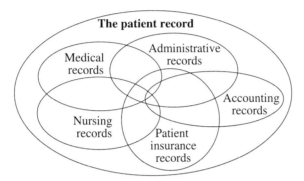

Figure 9.3 : Different views of a patient record

Objectives and Expected Benefits

Computer management of patient records stores a considerable amount of information in a minimal amount of space. The increased storage capacities and compression techniques are particularly significant for multimedia objects, which will play an increasingly important role in health care in the coming years (Figure 9.4).

Computerizing records can significantly improve their quality [Dick 1991]. A patient record stored on a computer is both more readable and more precise than a manual record. Automated entry procedures help to improve exhaustiveness (as regards a patient's various problems) and completeness. The number of medical subjects covered by physicians during a computer-assisted consultation increases significantly. The answer rate for questions asked systematically usually surpasses 95%, whatever the age or the computing experience of the physicians who use it [Degoulet 1990]. Data coming from different hospitals, or from consultations and hospitalizations, may be linked, ensuring improved continuity in health care.

Electronic records may be accessed immediately, 24 hours a day, and simultaneously by different users. Access times are reduced considerably. Computerized records facilitate data sharing and communication between the different partners in the health-care system (automatic printing of reports, access to clinical or biological data through the remote network, electronic transmission of medical or administrative information, etc.).

Once the information has been stored in an appropriate format, it may be displayed or searched according to the needs of the physician (tables, graphs, organized according to time, source, or problems). Automated, well-designed summaries have more informational value than traditional records and may improve the decision-making process.

Type of record	Traditional	Compu-terized
Information storage and communication		
- data integration (including multimedia data)	+	+++
- readability of the record	+	++
- coverage of all problems	+	++
- completeness (selected areas)	+	+++
- access	sequential	simultaneous
- availability of information	local	global
- remote access	0	+++
- chaining of treatment episodes	+	+++
- chaining of distributed records	0	++
Treatment and decision support		
- summaries, multiple abstractions	0	+++
- reminders, alarms	0	+++
- diagnostic or therapeutic suggestions	0	+++
- processing multimedia data	0	+++
Regrouping data		
- treatment evaluation	+	+++
- clinical, epidemiological research	+	+++
- management control, scheduling	0	+++
Training and education		
- ease of use of the record	+++	+
- formalization of the medical process	+	+++
- adherence to treatment protocols	+	+++
- connection to data/knowledge databases	0	+++
Security, protection		
- data security	+	+++
- confidentiality	++	+

Figure 9.4 : Comparison of traditional vs. computer-based records

Computerized records improve the quality of care (e.g., calculation of the dosage of a medication in a narrow therapeutic window, or radiotherapy planning). Reminders or alarms, which can be automatically triggered during data entry, are a precious aid to physicians [McDonald 1976, 1988; Rind 1995]. A practitioner assisted by a computer is less likely to forget simple medical gestures such as searching for contraindications for medication or preventive actions.

Computer-based records facilitate the regrouping of data for clinical research or care evaluation [Safran 1995]. Indeed, the intra- and inter-physician variability discussed in Chapter 3 is significantly reduced compared to that measured with traditional records. This regrouping is impossible, however, unless the data are stored in a coded format (as opposed to entering records as free text, which only allows limited processing). Searching a database for cases comparable to those of the patient may directly assist in the prognosis or in making medical decisions [Safran 1989, Chute 1992]. In some cases, they have an educational value, making concepts and procedures more explicit and requiring that knowledge be formalized [Weed 1991] (see Chapter 12).

Automatic connection procedures to documentary databases (e.g., searches for recent bibliographical references concerning a patient's problems) or knowledge bases (see Chapter 6) may be implemented. Computer-based medical records are both more accessible and better protected than traditional records. Technical means exist to guarantee their physical and logical protection (passwords, data encryption, etc.) and to ensure data confidentiality (see Chapter 15).

Despite these advantages, successful computerization is rare. Several kinds of difficulties complicate the process of putting records on the computer:

- Computerizing records requires complex medical data and knowledge modeling. The initial models, based on the linear organization of paper records, have rapidly proven to be insufficient.
- Medical terminology must be organized in complex dictionaries to achieve semantic coherence within pieces of distributed records [Cimino 1994, Rector 1994].
- Human problems are often underestimated, especially user interface problems, security, confidentiality, and the possible effect on the patient/physician relationship caused by the direct entry of the medical record in the patient's presence.
- The high cost of hardware, software, and access to communication networks are factors that inhibit the generalization of computer-based records.
- The training provided to health-care personnel to use computer systems is usually insufficient.

Modeling Medical Information

Modeling medical information includes two important steps:
- Defining the elements of the discussion (i.e., *standardizing* terminology). This entails the precise definition of each term used in the records, the semantic relationships between the terms, and the methods of response (see Chapter 5).

• Organizing the elements of the discussion in an appropriate model (i.e., the *structuring* stage).

How to Standardize Medical Terminology

This problem was discussed in Chapter 5. The principal classifications of medical terms that have been developed are not well adapted to their initial objective: codifying the causes of death for the WHO classification (ICD-10); key words in a scientific article for MeSH; and describing anatomical, pathological, or radiological lesions for SNOMED. They often prove insufficient as soon as a specialized medical discipline or a particular problem is discussed (encoding of symptoms and signs is usually incomplete). The development of more adapted terminologies, such as the READ codes developed by the National health Services in UK, raises the issue of their integration with other classification systems [NHS 1995, Brown 1998].

The SNOMED RT reference terminology or the UMLS metathesaurus can be used as a basis for creating a dictionary of terms used in a medical record, but actual usage is still experimental [Spackman 1997, Campbell 1998].

How to Structure Medical Records

Structuring may be defined as regrouping isolated elements to create more complex objects. Two types of structuring are often found in traditional patient records.

Source-Oriented Organization

Traditional patient records are *source-oriented* (or origin-oriented) to the information. Data obtained through interrogations (antecedents or symptoms), clinical examinations, complementary examinations, and diagnostic, therapeutic, and prognostic data are grouped together in different sections (Figure 9.5).

The diagnostic section is the most important since it integrates the maximum amount of data in order to make the right decisions. Evolutionary data are made up of subsets of the preceding sections.The contents of source-oriented records are greatly influenced by the speciality of the hospital service where the patient is located. There is a significant risk of neglecting the synthesis in favor of the analytic aspect and therefore neglecting certain problems that are not part of the service's speciality (for example, considering all risk factors, preventive measures, etc.).

Figure 9.6 illustrates a subset of a form used by ARTEMIS, a system for following hypertensive patients [Degoulet 1990, Lemaitre 1994]. Information is entered in the form of yes-no questions (e.g., spontaneous symptomatology yes=1, no=0), multiple-choice questions (e.g., physical activity or heart problems) or free text (e.g., description of symptoms).

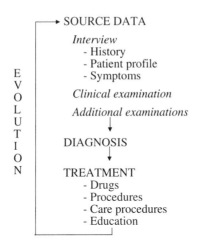

Figure 9.5 : Source-oriented medical record

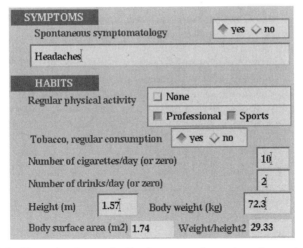

Figure 9.6 : Example of a standardized, structured questionnaire used to follow hypertensive patients

Problem-Oriented Organization

On the opposite track, the basic idea of *problem-oriented records,* proposed by Weed during the 1960s and illustrated in Figure 9.7, was to structure record contents according to a hierarchy whose root is a list of problems [Weed 1969]. The concept of problems is a larger one than the concept of diagnosis. It includes all diagnostic, therapeutic or surveillance conditions requiring special attention. A problem may be both a symptom and a diagnostic. Consider a patient who complains of headaches. The "headache" problem is added to the list of problems. The scanner shows an intra-cerebral mass. The problem becomes an intracerebral tumor. The headache symptoms are removed from the problem list, and attached to the preceding diagnostic.

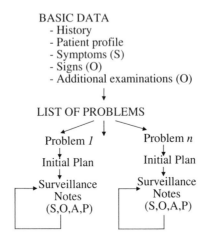

Figure 9.7 : Problem-oriented records. S: subjective, O: objective,
A: assessment, P: plan

The list of problems is established based on the collection of basic data (Figure 9.7). Problems are classified as active or inactive. For each active problem, an initial plan is established including the collection of new subjective (symptoms) or objective (signs) information, and therapeutic, drugs, follow-up or educational prescriptions. Surveillance notes are recorded problem-by-problem using the SOAP logic: S for subjective, O for objective, A for assessment and P for plan.

Structuring by problems presents two major advantages compared to source-oriented structuring: it emphasizes the importance of the problem list (the root of the tree) and forces the user to adopt an approach that is systematic by problem (*protocol*). However, it includes a certain number of constraints, in part due to the hierarchical model itself. Such a model is perfectly adapted when the different branches of the tree (i.e., the data associated with each problem) are independent, which is rarely the case for problems concerning the same patient. Evolutionary data are attached to elements (i.e., the problems) whose definitions are unstable over time. Furthermore, they are a function of the evolution of the profile of a patient's problems. In the end, the risk of redundant and/or inconsistent information is high. For example, a single beta-blocker may be prescribed for relatively distinct problems such as coronary insufficiency, arterial hypertension, or migraines. Inversely, a medication indicated for one problem may have adverse side-effects for another problem.

Searching for Underlying Structures

The two previous medical records models illustrate the complexity of the process of structuring medical information. They also show the limits to solutions historically associated with a linear conception of medical record storage (i.e., as in written documents). In both organizations, we can see that the concepts used change over time. A diagnosis or a problem established at time *t* may be considered as anterior to time *t* + 1 in the source-oriented organization, or as an antecedent or an inactive problem in the problem-oriented organization. The notion of an objective sign is in fact very subjective (for example, a large abdominal tumor).

By searching for better underlying structures, computing techniques let us envisage more complex structures, which make a clear distinction between the model for internal data representation and the view(s) that users may have of that data (i.e., the various surface structures). The theoretical objective is to design the underlying structure in the most general terms possible, and to establish bridges between the surface structures seen by the user (e.g., a source-oriented or a problem-oriented structure) and the underlying structure (Figure 9.8).

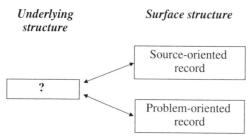

Figure 9.8 : Surface structure and underlying structures in a medical record

An example of such underlying structure is the *pragmatic record model* described in [Degoulet 1989]. Five pragmatic axes (S,T,O,R and M) are considered for building the model: the source of observation (or action), the time of observation (or action), the objects and their interaction, the receiver, and the methods used (e.g. to produce an observation or an action) (Figure 9.9). These axes are considered indispensable to the model but not necessarily sufficient. Other axes, such as the location (e.g. the place of utterance of an observation and the location of an action) or the intention (i.e. the goal) can be included and implemented in an extended version of the model.

In the pragmatic model, observations, actions or abstractions (i.e. concepts) are always considered in the context of their production. The source is one of the key elements of that context, since it partly or fully supports the act of interpretation. For a medical observation or action, the source can be a physician, nurse, patient, automatic device (e.g., a blood pressure monitor) or computer program like an expert system. For an abstraction (e.g., the concept of blood pressure or hypertension), the source can be an expert or a community of physicians. Several concepts are associated with the time axis, including events or points in time, intervals, periodic time and precedence (e.g., before, after). Events are represented as intervals with $t_1 = t_2$. Objects are

	Observation	Action	Abstraction
Example	SBP is 220mmHg	Furosemide 25mg *pid*	Hypertension
Source	Physician = x	Physician = x	World Health Organization
Time	$[t_1 - t_1]$	$[t_1 - t_2]$	$[t_1 - t_2]$
Object(s) and their interactions	(O_1) Patient = y (O_2) SBP = 220 mmHg (O_1) *has* (O_2)	(O_1) Patient = y (O_3) Furosemide = 25mg *pid* (O_1) *is–treated–by* (O_3)	(O_4) Disease = Hypertension (O_5) Vascular disease = disease category ($O4$) *is–a* (O_5)
Receiver	To whom it may concern	To whom it may concern	Medical community
Method	Manual BP measurement	Medical prescription	SBP >= 160 or DBP >= 95 mmHg

Figure 9.9 : Abstractions, actions and observations in the STORM pragmatic model. SBP: systolic blood pressure; DBP: diastolic blood pressure
(adapted from [Degoulet 1989])

defined by the classes to which they belong, by their behavioral properties inherited from classes and super-classes, and by their links (e.g., *is–a*, *has*, *caused–by*, *treated–by*, etc.) to other objects. The term receiver is applied in a broad sense. A receiver might be the addressee of a message, the patient to whom a drug is given, the community for which a concept is to be used (e.g. the medical community for the concept of hypertension), or a receptor in a biological structure. Methods express the way in which the relationships between the source, the objects and the receiver are obtained. For example, the method of blood pressure measurement might be auscultation, the automatic detection of sounds with a microphone or a Doppler method. The method of recording a symptom might be a patient interview by a physician or a computer.

Implementing Computerized Medical Records

The Software Environment

It is difficult to imagine computerizing a medical record without using a *database management system* (DBMS) (see Chapter 2). The choice of the most appropriate DBMS is not simple, however. The following points must be considered:

- the temporal dimension of medical data (i.e., the different visits of a single patient);
- the complexity of medical objects (e.g., plain language text or multimedia data); and
- the need to integrate medical data and knowledge to create decision-support systems (e.g., alarms, expert systems).

These difficulties explain why several teams, often in the teaching hospital environment, developed their own DBMS in the 1970s and 1980s rather than using commercial databases (hierarchical, network, or relational) [Goupy 1976, Barnett 1984, Degoulet 1986, Hammond 1986, McDonald 1988, Pryor 1988, Whiting-O'Keefe 1988]. The development of true object-oriented DBMS (OODBMS) or of object extensions to current relational DBMS may reverse this tendency, as these tools make it possible to model and manage complex medical information such as text and images as well as certain types of medical knowledge (e.g., semantic links between concepts, inheritance of properties or decision rules, etc.) [Doré 1995].

Most DBMS offer tools to create user interfaces. The trend is towards the use of user interface management systems (UIMS) independent of the DBMS, which operate in so-called client/server mode (see Chapters 1 and 2). Use of Internet-based interface manager is appealing because of the low cost and wide availability of these tools and their ability to integrate record manipulation functions with other tools such as access to knowledge bases or E-mail [Cimino 1995].

The theoretical advantages of a connection between the DBMS and an expert system or, more generally, a decision-support system, are obvious, be they to provide diagnostic, therapeutic or prognostic help, or training. Most connections are currently made by creating an interface between the DBMS and the expert system with a bidirectional transfer of information between the two programs.

Natural language in a computer-based record is often entered in the form of free-text comments with no particular computer processing, and stored in the database "as is". This method, where the surface structure of a medical record is identical to the underlying structure, offers fewer advantages over traditional record management. In any case, in restricted and well-conceptualized areas, automatic text analysis may improve the acceptability of computer-based medical records without leading to a significant loss of information. These automatic procedures that derive from natural language processing (NLP) techniques may be applied to the entry of a list of symptoms or problems, the analysis of a medical prescription, a radiological or pathological report or, in a much more distant future, a complete summary of the hospitalization [Baud 1992, Zweigenbaum 1995]. When a report in free text is analyzed during input, it becomes a particular surface structure of a standard, underlying structure such as a conceptual graph [Sowa 1984, Rassinoux 1995].

Processing complex objects, in particular signals and images, requires complementary programs (e.g. Web-based interfaces) as well as increased storage capacity for the database [Stewart 1998].

Patient Management Systems

Most general software and database tools must be combined to constitute a patient record management system that can be directly used by nonprogrammers. Figure 9.10 lists the functions traditionally included in a hospital department's system for managing patient records.

• Patient care and follow-up
 - Patient identification (permanent number)
 - Movements (admission, transfers, discharges)
 - Appointment scheduling
 - Health-care data entry (medical and nursing, during consultation and
    hospitalization)
 - Prescriptions (examinations, medications, interventions, training)
 - Generating reports and summary tables (by type of visit,
    by problem, by medical domain, etc.)
 - Decision support (alarms, diagnostic, therapeutic or prognostic
    suggestions, etc.)
• Health-care unit management
 - Communication
 - Activity reports (by diagnostics, type of activity, personnel, etc.)
• Research and training
 - Searching files by criteria
 - Access to bibliographical databases
 - Querying knowledge banks

Figure 9.10 : Sample functions of a patient record management system

It shows to what extent the architecture of such a system in a hospital is necessarily tied to the architecture of the underlying hospital information system (HIS).

 • In a centralized HIS architecture, all patient records will be stored in a physically unique database. Any HIS subsystems (e.g., laboratories, radiology) will feed this unique database.

 • In an HIS with a distributed architecture, the data in patient records is physically distributed between the subsystems. The record management system cannot access all information unless it can access a logical view of the full record and unless its DBMS provides access to different parts of the record. Although technologically interesting, this method may significantly increase response times and require the initiation of complex processes to guarantee data coherence and security. The risk of loss of privacy increases with the number of systems and therefore the number of entry ports into the network.

In a health-care network, security problems arise concerning the transmission of components of the patient's records between the various players in the network [Halamka 1997]. The integration of these components, required for decision-making, creates an additional problem concerning the "semantic" concordance of the terms used by the various players in the network. The *individual health card* (see smart cards, Chapter 1) may represent the electronic equivalent of a health-care personal paper record and may act as a link between the various players in the network [Beuscart 1996]. These cards must first be standardized concerning their contents and their readers, however. Public or private operators may also offer patients a secure service to maintain individual medical records, similar to a bank's service for financial deposits.

Hardware and Human Constraints

Installing a record management system requires the purchase and maintenance of expensive hardware that must be available 24 hours a day. Despite improvements in hardware reliability, availability rates above 99% are rarely achieved. In any case, procedures for downgraded operations must be established in case of a breakdown of the information system.

Ideally, information is entered directly by the person who created it (e.g;, physicians, nurses) (Figure 9.11). This data entry requires training of health personnel, made all the more difficult to organize because the turnover rate is high (e.g., medical students).

Information	Objective	Situation to avoid
Entry		
Who?	The person who manages the information	Whoever is available or who cannot refuse
When?	When the information is created	When it is possible
How?	Directly, without human intermediaries	Transcribed by an intermediary (e.g., a secretary)
Access		
For whom?	Those who create it	Those who manage it (computer programmers)
When?	Whenever they want it	If the programmers can or want to
How?	Directly, without any intermediaries	By intermediaries (programmers and/or statisticians)

Figure 9.11 : Methods for entering and accessing information

In most systems, data entry is performed indirectly, based on questionnaires from visits or reports dictated on cassettes, which must be transcribed by a secretary. This transcription extends the time required to update the records and is a potential source of error. Automatic voice recognition is not yet available for routine use. Significant results have been achieved in situations where a restricted vocabulary is sufficient (e.g., the semi-structured entry of pathological anatomy or radiology reports, or voice control of medical devices).

Interrogating and exploiting patient records usually requires dual training: in informatics for creating applications and in statistics for interpreting the results. This situation may be frustrating for users who, rightly, would rather avoid intermediaries.

Discussion and Conclusion

Computerizing medical records requires several steps: a detailed analysis of the structure of medical discourse, the selection of an appropriate model, the choice of an appropriate hardware and software infrastructure, and accounting for human and environmental factors (i.e., analyzing the needs, choosing a man-machine interface, and training all personnel concerned).

A clear distinction should be made between the surface structure of a medical record as seen by the user (organized according to the source or the problems) and the underlying structure as seen by the programmer. Although the first medical record management systems based their underlying structure on the surface structure (source- or problem-oriented record models), recent software bases models on more elaborate representations of data and knowledge.

Computer-based medical records are progressively replacing traditional records. They are also leading towards a greater integration of the entire health-care system. This integration with existing systems, databases, and expert systems under development represents one of the challenges facing computer-based records over the next decade.

Exercises

- *What are the objectives and expected benefits of computerizing patient records?*
- *What are the advantages of a computer-based record over a paper-based one?*
- *How to standardize and structure medical data in computer-based patient records?*
- *What are the advantages and disadvantages of source-oriented and problem-oriented organizations? How can computers improve structuring?*
- *Describe the minimal infrastructure required to implement a patient record.*
- *What are the principal difficulties that are expected when computerizing patient records?*
- *List a few of the problems concerning the distribution of patient record information in a health network, and discuss possible solutions.*

10
Physiological Signal Processing

Introduction

Several clinical situations lend themselves to the repetitive, closely grouped measurement of physiological parameters. These include recording electrical signals and measuring pressures, frequencies, volumes, flows, or temperatures. In general, physiological signals vary continuously over time. Data are captured using specialized captors that transform the input signal into an electrical signal that may be amplified and visualized on a cathode ray tube. Transforming the analog signal into digital data simplifies processing, storage, and transmission. This chapter briefly presents the objectives and bases for signal processing and describes a few significant examples.

Importance and Objectives

Information technology can play a role in all the steps involved in signal capture and processing, and help overcome human limitations in perception and interpretation. Digital processing improves signal quality, facilitates interpretation and provides direct help for making medical decisions. This assistance is all the more important given the large number of parameters to be surveyed, the high sampling frequency, and the extended duration of surveillance, as is usually the case in intensive care units.

- Coupling a computer system with specialized captors increases the perception capacity of the clinical technician. Although the human eye can visualize on-screen displays of significant variations in amplitude, shape or frequency, slow or complex variations, such as fluctuations in the amplitude and frequency of an EEG, may go unnoticed. Additionally, trace quality may be improved automatically, and noise may be separated from the actual signal.
- Computers can record signals over extended periods. Important signals, stored in digital form, may be redisplayed when needed. Automatic analysis of recorded signals, such as an EEG recorded during sleep or a Holter recording of an ECG over 24 hours, would not be practical without computer assistance.

- Digitizing signals facilitates their transmission. Contrary to analog signals, digital signals can be transmitted without distortion. Remote visualization of signals is used in *remote surveillance* systems. Signals may be transmitted between two hospital structures that may be geographically distant (teletransmission), which enables rapid consultation by an expert (or a program) and improves the quality of medical decisions.
- Automatic signal processing may be used to:
  - present data in multiple formats (e.g., tables, graphs);
  - automatically calculate new parameters (e.g., average pressure or frequency, tendencies);
  - compensate for human attention lapses by automatic alarm signals;
  - suggest actions; and
  - establish feedback loops (e.g., monitoring a perfusion).

Basic Signal Processing Concepts

Signal Acquisition

The process of capturing and processing signals corresponds to the general diagram in Figure 10.1. The signal is transformed into an electric current using a special device called a *transducer*. It is isolated and amplified, and then goes through analog to digital conversion (A/D) before being processed by the computer.

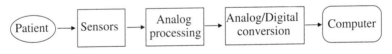

Figure 10.1 : The principle of signal processing

Sampling and Digitizing Signals

Before being processed by the computer, an analog signal must be digitized. This transformation is imperfect, but the information lost due to the conversion may be controlled by selecting the sampling frequency and the number of bits used for each sample. This process is illustrated in Figure 10.2.

The *precision* of a sample is a function of the number of bits N used to quantify each recorded point of the signal. For a given number of bits N, 2^N distinct values may be coded and samples taken are rounded to the nearest value that can be encoded in N bits. For a given sampling time T, we obtain a set of points that represent the digitized signal. The *sampling frequency* must be at least double the frequency of the signal being sampled (the Nyquist criterion). Thus, for an electrocardiogram, the sampling frequency recom-

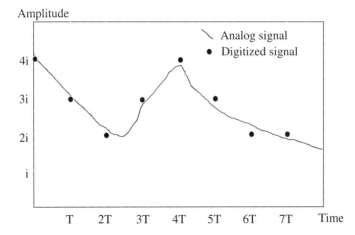

Figure 10.2 : Principle for analog/digital conversion. *T* is the sampling period; *i* represents the intensity scale of the signal, a function of the number of bits chosen to quantify the points

mended by the American Heart Association is 500 Hz (cycles/second). Figure 10.3 illustrates the loss of information that may occur when sampling frequencies are too low.

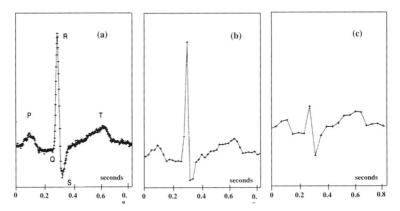

Figure 10.3 : The effect of sampling frequency. (a) Sampling at 500 points per second; (b) 50 points per second; (c) 25 points per second (adapted from [Gardner 1990a])

Basic Signal Processing Techniques

Numerous techniques are used in signal processing applications. They depend on the specifics of the problems to be solved and the goals to be achieved. Certain types of processes are nonetheless commonly used in clinical applications: signal enhancement, extracting pertinent traits and pattern recognition.

Signal Enhancement

Any recording of a physiological signal, such as the electrical activity of the heart, contains a *noise* component along with the signal itself. Noise may be due to the electronics in the measuring device, artifacts related to the patient's movements, or other signals recorded simultaneously. Averaging or digital filtering techniques can reduce the amount of noise and improve the *signal-to-noise* ratio.

Averaging several samples of the same signal can eliminate background noise if it does not correlate to the signal. This technique is illustrated in Figure 10.4.

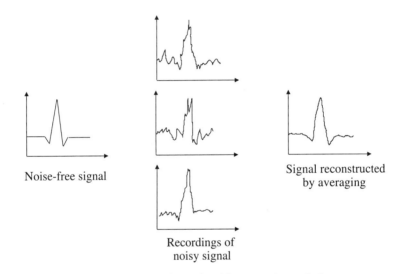

Noise-free signal

Signal reconstructed
by averaging

Recordings of
noisy signal

Figure 10.4 : Extracting a signal by averaging techniques

Digital filtering can reconstruct a signal by replacing the sample measured at time t by the weighted average of preceding samples (at times $t-1$, $t-2$, etc.) and recalculated measurements. According to the average weighting formula used, the contribution of some parasite frequencies can be reduced.

Extracting Relevant Traits

Some relevant information is not the direct result of a sample or recording of a signal. It then becomes necessary to transform the initial signal. For example, in order to interpret an EEG or an EMG, it must be separated into its different frequency components. The role of each wave form is analyzed using mathematical techniques such as Fourier transformations or spectrum frequency analysis.

Pattern Recognition

Relevant traits that have been identified may be submitted to a classification procedure that determines if the signal displays a problem known to the program. These procedures, called pattern recognition, often use automated learning techniques. They are based on mathematical models that may be very complex [van Bemmel 1997].

Sample Medical Applications

Medical applications make extensive use of signal analysis, particularly in the areas of screening, functional explorations, and intensive care. The following examples illustrate these possibilities.

Examples of Signal Analysis

ECG Analysis

The automatic analysis of ECGs is one of the oldest and most significant examples. A 1988 study in the United States showed that over 50% of the 100 million ECGs performed annually were analyzed by computers. Records may be stored in digitized form and analyzed locally or remotely after transmission to an interpretation center. Based on ECG sequences, programs can recognize and quantify complex QRS and P and T waves. R–R intervals are measured to detect certain rhythmic problems. Forms may be learned, stored, and then compared to the forms being observed. System performance for detecting certain disorders may approach that of cardiologists [Willems 1991, van Bemmel 1994].

Early detection of rhythm problems in intensive care units has become an essential element in reducing premature death by coronary thrombosis. Prolonged ambulatory ECG recording, using the Holter technique, can detect subtle cardiac rhythm problems. The signal is recorded on a magnetic tape and may be remotely analyzed and interpreted.

EEG Analysis

Extracting useful information from an EEG in a clinic is a difficult task. Current systems often offer assistance in interpreting the information rather than diagnostics, as is the case for ECGs.

Basic electroencephalograph techniques provide the different frequencies that make up the signal (e.g. alpha, beta, or gamma rhythms). Analysis of the potentials presented lets us study the cortex's responses to different stimuli (e.g., light, sound, tactile stimuli, or words). These analyses are useful for diagnosing sensorial deficits.

The study of sleep provides useful information for analyzing sleep-related problems such as insomnia or narcosis. The quantity of information is so large that manual analysis would be nearly impossible. Programs attempt to determine the stages of sleep and their sequences and duration, and to identify particular abnormal phenomena.

EEG analysis systems are currently not as well accepted by the medical community as the systems applied to ECG. The main reason for this reticence is the lack of consensus as to the method used to analyze these samples and the relevant information that characterizes these recordings.

Measuring Ambulatory Blood Pressure

Measurement of ambulatory blood pressure can be performed by an automatically inflating armband, and results are recorded by microphone or by the Doppler effect of arterial noise. Prolonged recording (e.g., for 24 hours) can be used to detect temporary variations of blood pressure, clarify the need for an antihypertensive treatment in the case of limited hypertension, or study the effect of a medication to precisely understand its effects and modify the dosage.

Intensive Care Monitoring

Intensive care environments are characterized by a high number of physiological parameters that must be monitored and the need for close supervision. Monitoring systems are particularly useful in the following applications:

- integrating signals from multiple sources: pressure (arterial, central venous, etc.) volumes, flows (cardiac, urinary, infusion), concentrations (glycemia), etc.;
- presenting information in the most appropriate form;
- interpreting variations over prolonged time periods;
- learning and recognizing profiles;
- triggering "intelligent" alarms. Sophisticated systems are able to recognize certain sampling *artifacts* such as moving an electrode. One signal can validate another. For example, the cardiac rhythm may be deduced from the ECG, as well as from blood pressure variations. An alarm is only triggered if the two measures agree.

The multiple sources of physiological signals require the development of standard hardware and software interfaces, such as the *Medical Information Bus* (MIB) standard published by the American IEEE association [Gardner 1990a].

It can be particularly interesting to integrate feedback loops, since the monitoring system operates on the "perception – interpretation – action" cybernetic model. For example, the infusion flow rate, the parameters of a ventilator, pacemaker, or renal dialysis device can be controlled.

Integration in Information Systems

The applications cited above become particularly interesting when they are integrated in the general information system. This step is required for monitoring in intensive care units. Patients in life or death situations must be under continual surveillance. A study carried out at the LDS Hospital in Salt Lake City, Utah, illustrates the variety of data used by a physician when making therapeutic decisions, and when patients are under surveillance in an intensive care unit (Figure 10.5).

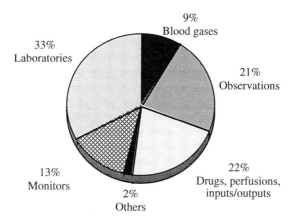

Figure 10.5 : Type of data used in intensive care units
(adapted from [Gardner, 1990a])

In order to solve this problem, systems must be able to capture physiological data, analyze that data, communicate with biology laboratories that may provide other information on the patient, synthesize this information and directly intervene in the decision.

Discussion and Conclusion

Digitizing physiological signals can improve the signal quality, facilitate their transmission over long distances and their interpretation, and provide direct assistance to decision-making. Information technology can improve patient surveillance by automatically triggering alarms and recording signals over extended periods.

The evolution of digital signal processing tools is moving towards their integration in general information systems. These authorize the use of information available on the patient's status, whatever the nature and source of the data. This evolution will lead to the development of decision support systems that are much more pertinent and useful to the physician. These systems are currently being developed in environments that offer tools for creating multimedia medical workstations.

Exercises

- *Cite the advantages of digitizing physiological signals.*
- *Understand how signal processing techniques can help normal clinical practice and discuss some examples.*
- *Explain the importance of integrating data coming from multiple sources to support clinical decisions.*

11
Medical Imaging Systems

Introduction

Imaging techniques occupy a growing part of the practice of medicine. They may intervene in the diagnostic, prognostic, or therapeutic decision-making processes. Medical images include radiological images (conventional radiography or tomography), nuclear-medicine, ultrasound, photography (used in cytology, pathology, dermatology, electrofluoresence or chromosome maps), films (endoscopy), functional images obtained through reconstruction (tomodensitometry, magnetic resonance imaging), or even simulations that create *virtual reality.*

We may distinguish two broad types of images:

- physical, optical, or electromagnetic (X-ray) images, which are analog and continuous by nature;
- mathematical images, digital by nature, generally corresponding to matrices of numbers, which generally represent the distribution of luminous intensities on all points of the image. Images obtained from tomographies are an example of this type.

Digitizing images, either from the start or at a later stage, facilitates their processing, storage, and remote transmission. These processes have developed considerably with the advent of efficient compression techniques and workstations with high storage capacity and sufficient computational power to implement the processing algorithms.

This chapter presents a summary of the objectives of medical imaging systems, the basis for image processing, and describes a few significant examples.

Importance and Objectives

Information technology can assist in all phases of gathering and processing medical images. A few examples illustrate the importance of image processing in medicine:

- Information technology directly generates certain types of images that could not be obtained otherwise such as computerized axial tomography (CAT scans), positron emission tomography (PET scans), and magnetic resonance imaging (MRI).
- Digital image processing may be used to:
  - improve image quality, compensate for imperfections in the image-generating system, and reduce noise;
  - identify quantitative parameters of clinical interest (measure distances, surfaces, densities, etc.);
  - propose interpretations (pattern recognition, calculate doses for radiotherapy, calculate courses); and
  - set up feedback loops (computer-aided surgical interventions).
- Image compression reduces the amount of storage required and the transmission time between distant sites.
- Storing digitized images on appropriate peripherals, such as magnetic disks or CD-ROM simplifies image management by reducing storage volumes and easing access and indexing.
- Remote transmission of digitized images within a hospital structure or between different structures allows several experts to rapidly consult the images for diagnostic or therapeutic decisions, and improves patient care (e.g., *teleradiology*, *telecytopathology*).

Image Acquisition Sources

Conventional radiology, using ionizing radiation from an X-ray source, remains the most prevalent method in radiology departments. It allows for short exposure times. The resulting image of superimposed organs crossed by X-rays is recorded on a radiographic film sensitive to X-rays. The image is digitized from these films. Digitized images may be produced directly (*digital radiology*) using phosphorous plates to replace conventional films.

Digital angiography displays the underlying vessels by subtracting undesirable structures (bones and organs) from the images. The first images, taken before the arterial or intravenous injection of the contrasting substance, are digitized. They are used to create a mask that will be subtracted from the images taken after the injection. Figure 11.1 illustrates the effects of the subtraction.

Computerized tomography also uses X-rays, but instead of being obtained directly, the image is rebuilt from the attenuation of the rays observed in different directions (Figure 11.2). Each image, from 256^2 to 512^2 pixels, corresponds to a cross-section of the appropriate part of the body. The exposure time is between 0.5 and 2 seconds per section.

Magnetic resonance imaging (*MRI*) techniques reconstruct images based on very different physical phenomena. The patient is placed in an intense

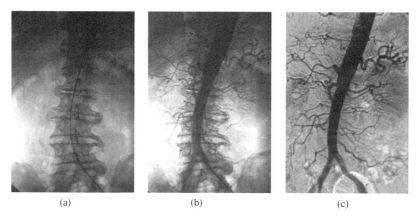

(a)   (b)   (c)

Figure 11.1 : Example of an image obtained by subtraction in digital angiography.
The image (c) is obtained by subtracting image (a) from (b). (Courtesy of
M. Kasbarian and J.M. Bartoli, Marseilles, France)

magnetic field, which orients the nuclei of atoms. Radio frequencies are
applied to make some atoms, such as hydrogen atoms, resonate. When the
emission stops, the atoms return to their initial state and emit a radio signal,
the intensity and duration of which depend on the biological characteristics
of the tissue that they cross. Without using ionizing radiation, MRI provides
images that depend on the metabolism and the characteristics of the tissues
through which they pass.

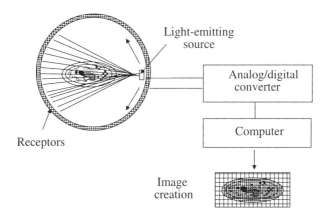

Figure 11.2 : The principle of computerized tomography

Ultrasounds are based on an acoustic probe that emits ultrasonic waves.
The probe also captures the reflected waves, and the probe's piezoelectric
crystals convert the acoustic echoes into electrical signals. The signals,
which come from several unidirectional paths, are digitized and processed.

They are stored in memory and transformed into a video signal that may be displayed on a screen as a two-dimensional image. The intensity of the video signal is proportional to the intensity of the echo.

Scintigraphic imaging is performed by injecting a radioactive isotope (marker) attached to a biological component (tracer) that has an affinity for a certain organ (e.g. the thyroid or the surrenal). The isotope emits radiation that is captured by a radiation-sensitive camera (e.g., a gamma camera). The recorded image sequence displays certain functions of the organ.

Figure 11.3 compares these different radiological imaging techniques, and some of their characteristics.

Type	Size (pixels)	Density (bits)	Ionizing radiation	3-D recon-struction	Tissue activity measure-ments
Conventional radiography	2048^2	12	Yes	±	No
Digital angiography	1024^2	12	Yes	Yes	No
Computerized tomography	512^2	16	Yes	Yes	No
Nuclear magnetic resonance imaging	256^2	12	No	Yes	Yes
Ultrasound	512^2	8	No	±	No
Scintigraph	128^2	8	Yes	No	Yes

Figure 11.3 : Characteristics of a few radiological imaging techniques

Several types of images outside the realm of radiology can also be digitized and processed. The images can be captured by video camera (endoscopy, microscopic pathological anatomy images, etc.) or from a photograph. True color processing is often necessary (e.g., quantifying the effect of a treatment on dermatological lesions).

Virtual reality is based on the creation of images based on the description of objects. These objects, set in three-dimensional space, may have colors and texture, and be subjected to various conditions of lighting, orientation and motion (e.g., the force of gravity). The user, placed in this virtual world, can even move around and interact with the objects.

Digitized Images

Spatial Coding

Images can only be processed by computers in the form of tables of numbers. A two-dimensional table (x,y) can represent a simple, two-dimensional image. Each element in the table corresponds to an elementary square surface or *pixel* (picture element). A three-dimensional table (x,y,z) is required to represent a volume. Each element in the table represents an elementary cube or *voxel* (volume element).

Pixel size defines the *spatial resolution*. The smaller the size, the less the digitizing process will lose information compared to the source image. Pixel sizes of less than $0,2 \times 0,2$ mm are necessary to maintain standard radiography quality.

Intensity Coding

The density of each pixel is coded on d bits. Eight-bit coding provides 256 coding levels, while 12-bit coding provides $2^{12} = 4096$ levels. This number determines the *contrast resolution*. If N and M represent the number of lines and columns in a table of pixels, the number of bits necessary to encode a two-dimensional image would be:

$$N \times M \times d \qquad (11.1)$$

For a black-and-white image, 256 levels correspond to 256 gray levels. For a color image, the same principle applies for each fundamental color chosen (red, green, and blue for RGB coding).

Temporal Coding

The *temporal resolution* measures the time required to create an image. A real-time application may require the creation of 30 images per second. At this speed, it is possible to obtain a clear image of an organ in movement, such as the heart.

Digitizing Images

In practice, digitizing systems frequently use square matrices corresponding to powers of 2 (256×256, 512×512, 1024×1024 pixels) with coding density from 8 to 24 bits. Figure 11.4 gives an example of digitizing an image containing 8×8 pixels with 10-bit coding.

A two-dimensional sequence of images over time requires a three-dimensional (3-D) table (x, y, t) and a 3-D sequence of images (volumes) requires a four dimensional table (x, y, z, t). Image sequences recorded over time may be coupled with physiological signals such as ECG (see Chapter 10). These images may occupy very large volumes (several hundred million bits). The JPEG (*Joint Photographic Experts Group*) standard is an image compression standard for still images, and MPEG (*Motion Picture Expert Group*) is used for moving pictures. Compression factors of 2 or 3 may be obtained without losing information compared to the digitized image, and factors of 8 to 10 may be obtained with only minimal loss.

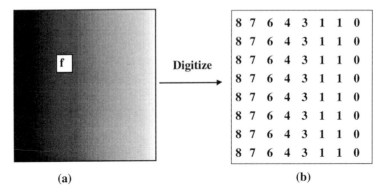

(a)   (b)

Figure 11.4 : The principle of digitizing images. (a) is the original image. Selecting the sampling window *w* leads to the matrix (b) obtained by quantifying on a scale of 10 gray levels (0 = white, 9 = black)

Basic Image Processing Principles

The Imaging Process

Image analysis involves a series of procedures (Figure 11.5) that constitute the imaging process. Each step in the process depends on the results of the preceding steps and on the operator's knowledge and experience. This may also be used to pilot the system and link the steps together.

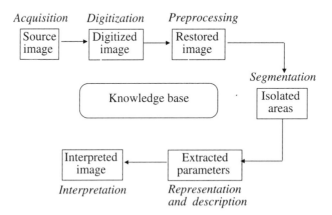

Figure 11.5 : The imaging process (adapted from [Gonzalez 1992])

The preprocessing phase improves image quality, and the segmentation phase isolates the elements that make up the image. Beyond these steps, we enter the realm of high-level vision. This involves extracting significant parameters of the image (e.g., the volume of a tumor or the degree of a stenosis) which play a role in its interpretation. The interpretation phase may lead to a diagnosis, a prognosis, or even a procedure as in robotics.

Image Preprocessing

The preprocessing phases eliminate imperfections related to the image generation system and reduce noise. The techniques used normally transform the value of each pixel in the original image into a new value obtained by a mathematical function. They improve the visibility of certain anatomical structures.

Noise Reduction

Image noise in conventional radiology or nuclear medicine is primarily due to the random nature of the attenuation of X-rays by tissue or the emission of gamma rays. It causes a reduction in contrast. Different filtering techniques can reduce this noise. The smoothing method recalculates the density of each point according to the density of the adjacent points.

Modifying Image Contrast

Calculating the histogram of an image creates a representation of the number of pixels for each gray level (density) of the image. Figure 11.6 shows a sample histogram of Figure 11.4.

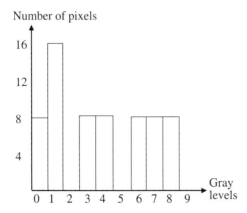

Figure 11.6 : Histogram of the image digitized in Figure 11.4

Analysis of the histogram makes apparent the distribution of gray levels in an image and helps judge the quality of the digitization. If the histogram is centered on density values that are too weak or too strong, the strong or weak values, respectively, are lost, and the image has too little or too much contrast. Operations to transform the histogram of an image may improve the contrast (and the visual perception) in particular gray areas.

Geometric Operations on Images

Geometric operations perform block moves on an image and generate an unvarying output image after a translation or a rotational movement. It is also possible to enlarge a region to analyze details.

Segmentation

The segmentation phase isolates elements in the image (organs, vessels, microscopic cells, etc.). Different techniques are used. The methods are usually based on identifying differences in density around the edges of the desired object. The *threshold method* keeps only pixels whose intensity is between upper and lower limits.

The *outline isolation* method plots the levels of a digitized image to show the structure and the shape of the organ, as shown in Figure 11.7 obtained from a thyroid scintigraph.

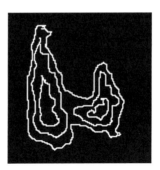

Figure 11.7 : Isolated outlines of a thyroid gland

Subtracting two images shows details that are difficult to see on the original image (the case of digitized angiography) or analyzes variations over time.

Three-dimensional images can be reconstructed from layered cross sections of certain images, such as those from tomodensitometry or MRI. Projecting shadows on the surfaces of reconstructed objects improves visibility, as seen in Figure 11.8 obtained from MRI images of the heart [Meinzer 1990].

Extracting Parameters

This technique can be used when measuring a surface or a volume (e.g., cardiac volume, the volume of a tumor), quantifying shrinkage (e.g., vascular

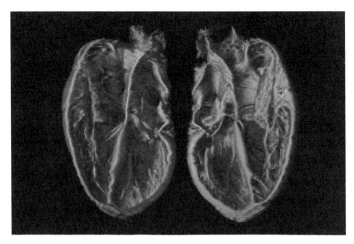

Figure 11.8 : Reconstitution of a three-dimensional image from cross-sections obtained by MRI (courtesy of H.P. Meinzer and U. Engelmann, Heidelberg, Germany)

stenosis), evaluating a texture (e.g., bone density) or counting elements (e.g., cells or calcifications).

Image Interpretation

Automatic computer interpretation of images presents complex research problems. It requires knowledge of several disciplines, in particular anatomy and pathological anatomy. The structures and parameters identified must be compared to known structures and then classified. A combination of images obtained using different image capturing methods or clinical or biological data is often required to propose an automatic diagnosis.

Sample Medical Applications

Quantifying the Degree of a Vascular Stenosis

Treatment of vascular stenosis was revolutionized by endoluminal dilation techniques, which avoided complex surgery. Therapeutic indication and remote patient care require a precise quantification of the arterial lesions, which may be performed automatically or semiautomatically as shown on figure 11.9 [Cherrak 1997].

Identifying Chromosomes

Identification of chromosomes when determining the karyotype uses pattern recognition techniques. The 23 pairs of human chromosomes may be identified by their relative size and the position of their centromere.

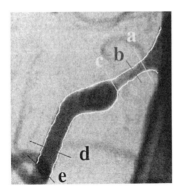

Symbolic description:

Dilatation (length 11% of total length)
 (aspect non-centered)
Stenosis (length 27% of total length)
 (degree 61%)
 (aspect centered)
 character irregular)
 (position troncular)
Dilatation (length 28%)
 (aspect centered)
Normal (length 34%)

Figure 11.9 : Automatic stenosis detection and quantification in a renal arteriography (courtesy of MC. Jaulent and associates, Paris, France)

The image of a cytological preparation is digitized, and its variations in density are analyzed. After identifying each chromosome, the computer tries to group them in pairs. Several methods have been used for these tasks. The Mendelsohn method is based on the following principle (see Figure 11.9). The axis of each chromosome is determined, and the sum of its pixel densities is calculated in a direction perpendicular to that axis. The profile of the chromosome is thus obtained, and the minimum density for that profile is determined by the position of the centromere. The length of the profile and the position of the minimum classifies the chromosome.

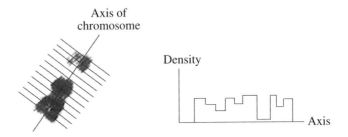

Figure 11.10 : Analysis of chromosomes, determination of the profile

Computer-Aided Surgical Techniques

The objective of computer-aided surgery is to facilitate certain surgical techniques (e.g., puncture, positioning a prosthesis, or inserting a probe).

The techniques used are part of the classical robotics loop: perception – reasoning – action" [Cinquin 1996]. The perception step concerns the acquisition of the necessary images, often using several methods. Reasoning develops a model of the patient and simulates the procedure. Finally, the medical–surgical procedure is carried out. The computer can supply passive assistance (it compares what the surgeon is doing with what was planned, and eventually triggers alarms), semiactive assistance (the strategy is constrained by automated tools) or active assistance (some tasks are directly assigned to the robot). Figure 11.10 shows an example of robotic guidance used in stereotactic surgery and developed by the team of J. Demongeot and Ph. Cinquin at the Grenoble University Hospital in France.

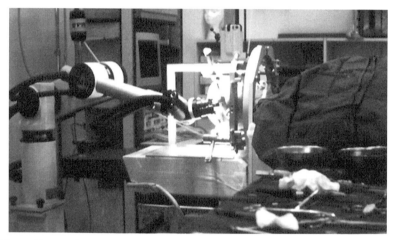

Figure 11.11 : Computer-aided surgical gesture (courtesy of J. Demongeot and Ph. Cinquin, Grenoble, France)

Virtual Reality

Virtual reality attempts to make the artificial seem as lifelike as what is real, if not more so. Flight simulation is one of the oldest virtual reality applications, enabling pilots to practice flying aircraft without risking equipment loss or passenger lives.

Two major techniques are used to represent images in three dimensions. Holography presents all the possible views of a scene in a single plane of modulated light. It requires very high resolution images that are difficult to counterfeit. The perception of 3-D images may be obtained using a headset with special glasses or a video helmet, by providing the eye with a slightly shifted image that corresponds to normal binocular vision. The rapid processing of digitized images lets the user associate head movements with simultaneous movements in the field of vision. This technique considerably improves the rendering of projected scenes as well as the coupling with audio or olfactory signals. *Data gloves*, sensitive to finger movements, may be used as an input peripheral to let the user move around in the virtual world. It is easy to imagine the potential of these techniques for teaching medicine (anatomy, for example) or simulating surgical procedures.

Imaging Management and Communication Systems

Various types of systems integrating complex functions are currently appearing. The technological solutions on the market can integrate video displays and digital processing functions in a single workstation [Meinzer 1996]. They foreshadow future applications of cooperative medicine (discussed in Chapter 8 on health-care networks). In the more limited framework of this chapter on image management, we can differentiate two types of situations:

Tele-expertise

Exchanging information requires a high degree of interactivity and may necessitate access to information already stored in patient records and also may require storage of the information exchanged. In this case, the techniques used include the transmission of voice, digitized images, and also video techniques and videoconferencing, eventually integrated in a single workstation. The classic example of this type of activity involving image transmission is consulting an expert in pathological anatomy.

PACS

Images are integrated in a system to manage the patient's "image" records. The system must provide archiving of and rapid access to images. The PACS (*picture archiving and communication system*) is designed to manage these tasks. Digital image management becomes part of the development of the hospital information system [Ratib 1994, Engelmann 1995].

These computing systems archive, process, communicate, and display all medical images produced by one or several institutions. The image archiving and communication systems so designed offer the following advantages:

- they can store digital images without the risk of loss or deterioration of their contents;
- they provide quick and easy access to all images for all authorized individuals; and
- they enable local processing (for both image production centers and users).

From an economic standpoint, they help reduce personnel, hardware, and maintenance costs [Enning 1994].

The PACS currently under development integrate different methods for obtaining images (digital radiographs, digitized angiographs, scanners, MRI, etc.). The large volume of information represented by these digitized images requires the installation of appropriate image servers, such as high-capacity magnetic disks for recent images and CD-ROM juke boxes for older images (see Chapter 1). The transmission of images and related information (e.g., type of film or incidence) requires the selection of compression and communication standards such as the ACR/NEMA DICOM standard.

Two types of display stations may be distinguished:

• processing and analysis stations with high resolution screens, often more than one for simultaneously viewing image sequences, and specialized processing chips; and

• care unit display stations, with reduced processing capacity.

Figure 11.12 illustrates a sample image display program called Osiris, developed at the Geneva Cantonal University Hospital, Geneva, Switzerland [Ligier 1994].

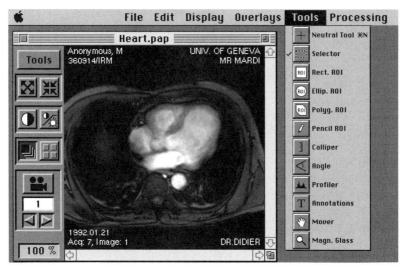

Figure 11.12 : Sample image display in the health-care unit using the Osiris® program (courtesy of O. Ratib and associates, Geneva, Switzerland)

Discussion and Conclusion

Digitizing medical images offers interesting possibilities:

• For daily patient care. Within a private practice or a radiology service, digitization offers useful treatments, while elsewhere it offers increased image communication facilities.

• For research and widening of medical knowledge.

• For developing simulation and training tools.

It seems likely that this sector of activity is at the beginning of a period of rapid expansion. In the long term, all images that are produced will be digitized and processed.

The integration of imaging systems in information systems both inside and outside hospitals requires standards for compressing, storing, and transmitting images. It also requires the installation of multidisciplinary teams

grouping image producers (e.g., radiologists or biologists) computer specialists, and clinical technicians.

Exercises

- *Cite the advantages of digitizing medical images.*
- *Describe the imaging process.*
- *Cite a few basic image processing techniques.*
- *Define virtual reality and its potential interest in medicine.*
- *Define an image communication and archiving system (PACS) and its importance in a hospital information system or a health-care network.*

12

Medical Decision Support Systems

Introduction

The practice of medicine requires the physician to constantly make multiple decisions that are logically related for a given patient. Computers can provide direct or indirect assistance in making these decisions. Hospital information systems (see Chapter 7) and systems for managing patient records (see Chapter 9) are part of the indirect assistance. Simplified access to patient records (e.g., laboratory data) and analytical presentations of data (e.g., reports or summary tables) can also help make decisions and avoid unnecessary or dangerous ones. This may involve providing access to data specific to a given domain, such as bibliographical databases or medical or legal knowledge bases (see Chapter 6).

This chapter deals with the more direct assistance that computer systems can provide when making decisions about a patient. They apply medical knowledge to the specific problem of a given patient and suggest solutions that offer the best cost–efficiency ratio. On the one hand, this method requires integrating reasoning mechanisms (such as those defined in Chapter 4) into the health-care management system and, on the other hand, evaluating and verifying their practical or theoretical effects. It requires precise knowledge of the actions performed by health-care personnel, the process for providing health care (see Chapter 4), the needs that have been expressed, and the current and future possibilities of decision support systems.

Although problems often appear to be identical on a theoretical level, this does not hold true in practice. The assistance expected from a decision support system depends on the clinical context and on the type of users. A prolonged fever is treated differently in an internal medicine service than in an intensive care unit. A student does not have the same expectations as an experienced physician.

Characteristics of Decision Support Systems

Types of Support

Medical decision support systems follow the general nature of medical interventions: predict (predictive medicine), prevent (preventive medicine), heal (curative medicine), or at least comfort (medical assistance). To achieve this goal, the patient's particular situation must be considered (diagnosis or prognosis) and possible strategies evaluated. Two types of decision support systems may be distinguished based on this approach:

- Systems to better understand a patient's state (i.e., *what is true*). They basically concern decisions for diagnosis or prognosis. They attempt to reduce the uncertainty of the patient's current or future situation. These systems must consider several sources of medical knowledge from various disciplines: epidemiology, semiology, pathology, physiology, anatomy, etc.

- Systems that attempt to suggest the best strategy (i.e., *what must be done*). Which additional tests should be performed? Which changes in daily routine should be made, what medication or treatment should be suggested? What is the best way to inform the patient of his condition? These systems must include financial and ethical considerations.

In practice, systems are usually a mixture of both. It is difficult to separate the therapeutic side of a problem from the diagnosis, and it can be very helpful to provide useful additional information concerning the patient or knowledge.

Types of Intervention

Passive Systems

Most decision support systems operate in a *passive mode*. The physician must explicitly make a request to the system. The physician describes the patient's case and waits for the system's advice. Two approaches are used, depending on the information supplied and the advice required:

- In a *consultant system,* the user supplies information on the patient's state, and the system provides diagnostic or therapeutic advice. MYCIN, developed by E. Shortliffe and assistants at Stanford University, is a typical consultant system [Shortliffe 1990].

- In a *critical system,* the user supplies information on the patient and on the physician's planned strategy (therapeutic and/or investigative). The system makes a critique of the physician's proposals. The ATTENDING system, developed by P. Miller at Yale University, New Haven, Connecticut, is a good example. It provides a critique of an anesthetic plan provided by the specialist for a given patient (e.g., anesthetics chosen, induction, administration) [Miller 1986a].

Semiactive Systems

Semiactive decision support systems are invoked automatically. They provide information and generally accepted knowledge and procedural rules. The system plays the role of a watchdog. In this category, we find

- *Automatic reminder systems* which supervise the care provider's actions [McDonald 1976]. They help avoid redundant examinations and prescription errors (by recognizing dosage errors and listing contra-indication for drugs and significant interactions). They make it easier for the medical team to follow pre-established protocols.
- *Alarm systems* signal changes in the patient's state. This may mean flagging abnormal values (e.g., biological or physiological parameters) or abnormal modifications (e.g., an abrupt rise or fall of a given parameter).

Active Systems

Active systems, which are triggered automatically, can provide advice adapted to a particular patient. They can automatically make decisions without the intervention of the physician. This may concern orders for additional examinations based on health protocols, therapeutic examinations (e.g., automatic control of a transfusion by a closed-loop system), supervision (e.g., intelligent control of the parameters of a ventilator, a dialysis monitor, or a pacemaker), or surgical assistance (see Chapter 11).

Types of Knowledge

Decisions require the application of specific knowledge to a clinical case (Figure 12.1) [Degoulet 1995]. At least three types of information are involved in the decision making process (see Chapter 4):

- *Observations* that may be supplied to the decision support system for making inferences (see Chapter 4).
- *Academic knowledge*, normally contained in books and medical journals (i.e., knowing that).
- *Experience* acquired in medical practice (i.e., knowing how). This may be medical behavior (such as knowing how to ask questions or to reassure), or medical know-how (such as knowing how to examine a patient or perform a medical procedure). Experience also helps the physician recognize and benefit from similar cases.

These different types of knowledge are interrelated in the decision-making process. Academic knowledge and experience determine the methods used to gather information and the quality of observations. Experience can confirm and add to academic knowledge. Recording observations such as preliminary diagnoses and decisions in medical records is indispensable for automated learning and verifying decision rules.

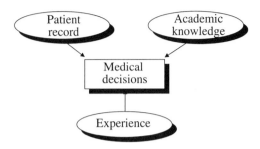

Figure 12.1 : Basis for medical decisions

Methodological Basis of Decision Support Systems

Decision support systems utilize a broad variety of methods besides simple algorithms. Each of these methods uses particular means of reasoning (Figure 12.2).

Method	Reasoning	Explanations	Learning
Mathematical models	Algorithmic	No	No
Statistical & probabilities	Inductive	Limited	Automatically by induction
Expert systems	Deductive, abductive	Yes	Difficult, supervised
Neural networks	Inductive	No	Supervised or automatic

Figure 12.2 : Methods for decision support systems

Using Mathematical Models

Mathematical models have been available for several decades for describing complex biological or physiological systems (e.g., hemodynamics, the effect of ionizing radiation on tissue, or pharmacokinetics). These models may directly assist in making decisions, either in a passive mode (analyzing the consequence of the variation of one or several parameters) or in an active mode (automatic controls).

Statistical Methods

The statistical methods of interest here are mainly based on multidimensional classification techniques. A patient is assigned to a therapeutic or diagnostic class according to the values of certain parameters x_i. A learning sample is created, from cases where the diagnostic, prognostic, or therapeutic decision has been made to find the discriminatory values and to estimate the values and their coefficients a_i. We may apply it to the given patient's case once the decision equation has been established.

Examples of statistical tools include multiple regression and discriminant analysis. They may be used for diagnostic (e.g., discriminant analysis), prognostic or therapeutic classifications (e.g., multiple regression).

Take the following model as an example:

$$f(D) = a_1 x_1 + a_2 x_2 + \dots + a_n x_n \tag{12.1}$$

for two medical diagnoses (appendicitis and salpengitis) and three signs and symptoms (abdominal rigidity written AR; pain in the right lower quadrant written PRLQ; and pain in the left lower quadrant, written PLLQ). We shall use the following discriminating equations:

$$f(\text{appendicitis}) = 4 \cdot \text{AR} + 10 \cdot \text{PRLQ} - 10 \cdot \text{PLLQ} \tag{12.2}$$

$$f(\text{salpingitis}) = 3 \cdot \text{AR} + 5 \cdot \text{PRLQ} + 5 \cdot \text{PLLQ} \tag{12.3}$$

For a patient with pain in both iliac fossa without any guarding symptoms, we would obtain:

$$f(\text{appendicitis}) = 0 + 10 - 10 = 0 \tag{12.4}$$

$$f(\text{salpingitis}) = 0 + 5 + 5 = 10 \tag{12.5}$$

Therefore, the proposed diagnosis is salpingitis.

Probability-Based Systems

Probability-based systems essentially use Bayes' formula and decision theory (see Chapter 4 and Appendix B). The *a posteriori* probability of observing a diagnosis Di when a sign S is present $P(D_i|S)$ depends on the *a priori* probability of the diagnosis and that of observing the sign when the diagnosis is present (*conditional probability*):

$$P(D_i|S) = \frac{P(D_i) \cdot P(S|D_i)}{\sum_{i=1}^{n} P(D_i) \cdot P(S|D_j)} \tag{12.6}$$

Bayes' approach accounts for positive and negative signs, and performance is usually acceptable. The concordance with experts often exceeds 70%, and results improve as the number of cases in the learning base increases. Without the case database, the estimation of *a priori* probabilities and conditional probabilities can initially be provided by experts and then replaced by real probabilities calculated on the case database as it develops.

Bayes' method has three inherent limitations that are more difficult to overcome: the exhaustiveness of decisions (the sum of the probabilities of the diagnostics D_i equals 1); the exclusiveness of decisions; and the independence of signs and symptoms. An "other" class can be created to cover all cases. This class, heterogeneous by nature, should only represent a small percentage of all decisions (contrary to the previous example). The exclusivity of decisions rarely corresponds to reality (one patient may have several diagnoses). Nevertheless, it is always possible to create an additional diagnostic class that combines two diagnostics. Two signs are rarely independent of one another, and the degree of linkage varies according to the diagnosis. It is therefore important to check these linkages in the case database and, if two signs appear linked, keep only the most significant ones. Mathematical techniques have been proposed to account for some interactions.

Artificial Intelligence and Expert Systems

Artificial intelligence (AI) is "the study of ideas and techniques which make computers intelligent" [Winston 1992]. This field has two objectives:

- the practical objective of making computers more useful and
- the theoretical one of better understanding the mechanisms of human intelligence.

AI is situated at the intersection of various disciplines: computer science, linguistics, cognitive psychology, and epistemology. One of the major repercussions of artificial intelligence has been the development of expert systems — computer programs that use specialized knowledge and inference mechanisms to obtain high performance levels in specialized domains.

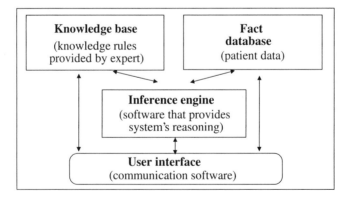

Figure 12.3 : General architecture of an expert system

Knowledge in expert systems is generally supplied as rules or frames (see Chapter 4). The *knowledge base* is separated from the base containing the problem-related data or the *factual base* of the system that creates the inferences, the *inference engine* (Figure 12.3). Expert systems use either classical logic or logic than can manage uncertainty. They allow heuristic reasoning. MYCIN was the first in a long list of applications developed in the 1970s and 1980s [Shortliffe 1976, Fieschi 1986, Winston 1992, Miller 1994].

For well-defined problems where no algorithmic solutions are available, the existence of experts makes possible the creation of knowledge bases (Figure 12.4). The expert systems are nonetheless limited by the difficulties involved in building and maintaining the knowledge base. Several disciplines contribute to this knowledge (e.g., anatomy, physiology, pathology), often inconsistent or contradictory. Knowledge is not easily split into the rules or structured objects required by expert systems. Without a sensory organ, expert systems start from information that the user has already interpreted. They have difficulty integrating new types of knowledge into existing knowledge (metaknowledge) and perceiving when they are leaving their area of expertise. Limited reasoning mechanisms (e.g., deduction and abduction) do not always correspond to those used by specialists, which are often more associative and intuitive.

Indications
- Human expertise might be lost
- Human expertise is scarce
- Expertise is needed in many locations
- Expertise is needed in hostile environments
- Task solution has a high payoff (usefulness, efficiency, etc.)

Feasibility
- Tasks require cognitive skills
- Specialized knowledge
- No algorithmic solution
- Moderately complex tasks
- Knowledge relatively static
- Genuine experts exist
- Experts are better than amateurs

Limitations
- Mixed representation schemes
- Knowledge is infinite
- Knowledge is contradictory or inconsistent
- The computer is blind; it needs an intermediary
- It is difficult to extend beyond the microworlds of the expert systems
- Reasoning is limited (deduction, abduction)
- Difficult to validate knowledge

Figure 12.4 : Indications, feasibility, and limitations of expert systems
(adapted from [Waterman 1986])

Neural Networks and Connectionist Systems

Although the first connectionist systems were designed in the 1940s and 1950s, their rapid growth and practical applications are recent (since the late 1980s) and resulted from the development of increasingly powerful microprocessors able to simulate their behavior. These were soon replaced by networks of microprocessors that led to the first hardware implementations (connectionist machines).

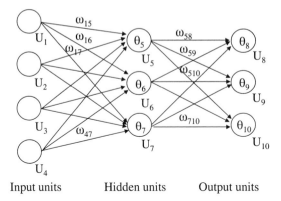

Input units   Hidden units   Output units

Figure 12.5 : General architecture of a neural network

The architecture of connectionist systems is inspired by the structure and operation of the human brain, hence the name *neural network*. Figure 12.5 illustrates one possible architecture of a neural network. The network is made up of nodes or *formal neurons, U_i,* linked by arcs. Information is propagated from nodes which form an input layer, through one or a series of hidden intermediate layers of neurons, to nodes that form the output layer. The stimulation level of a neuron equals the sum of the stimuli (the connection points ω_{ij}) of the related neurons. If this sum exceeds a certain activation threshold θ_i, the neuron stimulates other neurons connected to it. The relative weight of these connections and the stimulation thresholds is calculated by learning from cases supplied to the input layer.

The first practical applications of neural systems were form recognition systems (for recognizing characters, voices, image contours, etc.). They are well suited to diagnostic classifications when a sufficient case database is available. The input layer of the network represents the symptoms and the output layer represents the diagnoses.

Implementing Decision Support Systems

Despite considerable effort developing decision support systems, the actual number of operational systems in clinical practice remains small. The problems involved with their installation, along with the more specific ones of a particular method (see above), should be emphasized.

The User Interface

The quality of the user interface is a key factor for the system's acceptance. Physicians are not often attracted by computer terminals. The ergonomics of the interface must be carefully designed so that the system can be used in normal working conditions. The system should be easy to use and the learning curve minimal (see Chapter 2). Data entry required for the decision support system should not be redundant with the entry of patient records. In any case, the information supplied must be verified to ensure the reliability of the decision support system.

Knowledge Acquisition and Representation

Most decision support systems need a reliable base of medical records. This base is used to create the *a priori* and *a posteriori* probabilities of the diagnoses, to record decisions and their results, and to validate the knowledge. The base requires a logistical infrastructure that is difficult to implement: on-site data entry, connection to the management systems of ancillary systems to avoid re-entering information, training personnel to use the software, etc. (see Chapter 9).

Knowledge-based systems, like expert systems, rely on the availability of experts recognized in their field. The development of software to enter and update knowledge is difficult. Experts may have contradictory and/or fluctuating opinions. Knowledge bases should ideally be complete (i.e., all possible cases should be anticipated and the necessary knowledge should be available) and should not be contradictory. All knowledge cannot be represented, in particular knowledge concerning medical know-how and behavioral knowledge [Degoulet 1995].

Evaluating and Validating Systems

The evaluation of a decision support system presents methodological problems pertaining to the validity of the knowledge base, the methods of reasoning (the inference engine), and the validity of the proposed solutions [Fieschi 1990] . Knowledge of a reference decision is necessary to evaluate the proposals of the decision support system. Standard solutions (a *gold standard*) frequently do not exist in medicine. Experts do not always agree on the solution to be chosen, which considerably complicates evaluating the decision support system.

In any case, a statistical evaluation (where results are supplied as percentages obtained on a sample) is not always satisfactory. How does one judge a system that agrees with human experts 95% of the time and disagrees 5% of the time for cases where a patient's life may be affected by a wrong decision?

Integrating Decision Support Modules in Information Systems

Hospital information systems (HIS) have traditionally been developed around patient databases for the various medical and administrative services to find the information in a format that corresponds to their requirements. In the past, efforts to integrate medical knowledge in the HIS were limited. Traditional systems were usually administrative and logistical tools for managing patients rather than systems for managing medical data. Global patient care requires the integration of five types of information:

- patient data;
- medical knowledge;
- communications between health-care personnel;
- informing patients; and
- hospital administration and logistical data.

In the future, an HIS must cover all these areas, in particular theoretical and practical medical knowledge.

Sample Decision Support Systems

The numerous systems developed concern all the medical specialities. Here we will illustrate only a few of the major methods used and important experiments.

Pharmacokinetics and Assistance in Calculating Dosages

The concept of a population's pharmacokinetics was introduced in the early 1970s by Sheiner and colleagues [Sheiner 1972]. A pharmacokinetic model lets us represent and quantify a drug's various metabolism phases (e.g., absorption, diffusion, transformation in active and inactive metabolites, and elimination). When such a model is possible, the average and the distribution of the model's parameters are estimated for the target population that might receive the drug. When a potential patient appears, the uncertainty concerning the value of his own kinetic parameters corresponds to the variability between individuals in the target population. Measuring the patient's biological parameters reduces the uncertainty of the kinetic parameters. The model may be used to adjust the dosage. The clinical use of this method is particularly important for medication with a narrow therapeutic window (i.e., the interval of the optimal dosage is small and there is a high risk of inefficiency or overdose) and for which a simple pharmacokinetic model has been established (e.g., lithium, certain antibiotics or cytoxic agents, and antiarhythmics).

Assistance in Diagnosing Acute Abdominal Pain

The best known system, developed by de Dombal and colleagues, has been evaluated in various situations [de Dombal 1979]. The data in Figure 12.6 illustrate the importance of this method. In both of the experimental hospitals involved, the evaluation shows that physicians without the decision support system make the correct diagnosis less frequently than physicians with the system. Complications (appendix perforation) and unnecessary surgical procedures (laparotomies) are also less common when the system is used.

	Participating hospitals	
	Leeds (5,000 cases)	Edinburgh (2,500 cases)
First diagnosis correct		
without the system	45%	55%
with the system	63%	77%
Perforative appendicitis		
without the system	36%	25%
with the system	<10%	<10%
Unnecessary laparotomies		
without the system	24%	18%
with the system	10%	10%

Figure 12.6 : Evaluating the impact of a decision support system on health care
(adapted from [de Dombal 1979])

Diagnoses in Internal Medicine: INTERNIST and QMR

The most demonstrative examples of *diagnostic* assistance are the INTER-NIST/CADUCEUS/QMR systems initially developed by H. Pople, J. Myers, and R. Miller at the University of Pittsburgh, Pennsylvania [Miller 1982]. The work that led to these systems has greatly influenced research in the area. The system covers approximately 80% of internal medicine and uses a knowledge base of 4,500 signs and symptoms and 600 diseases. Each disease is described by approximately 80 signs. An expert has assigned two numbers to each pertinent sign for a given disease:

- a number between 1 and 5 that represents the frequency of the association;
- a number between 0 and 5 that represents the evocative power of the sign for the given disease.

A third number between 1 and 5 is associated with each sign. It represents the need to explain the sign in the final diagnosis. A value of 1 represents a sign that may appear in healthy individuals and where an explanation is not important. A value of 5 is assigned to a sign that must be explained by the final diagnosis.

Given the signs presented by the patient, the system determines a score to classify the various diagnostic hypotheses, knowing that they are not mutually exclusive. The performance of the system, as measured by clinical cases from the New England Journal of Medicine, was comparable to that of an expert. Although this development is exemplary concerning knowledge engineering, in practice the system is difficult to use for several reasons such as the time required to consult the system. Another version of the system, called QMR (Quick Manual Reference), is available on microcomputers [Miller 1986b].

Assistance in Chemotherapy: ONCOCIN

The ONCOCIN system, developed at the Stanford Oncology Clinic at Stanford University, California, and designed to help prescribe chemotherapy for cancer patients, illustrates the problems involved in implementing complex protocols in the area of therapeutic assistance [Hickam 1985, Shortliffe 1986]. It helps to identify and select the therapeutic protocols that may be applied to a patient, determine chemotherapy doses, and manage and supervise treatment. The system, which was developed on workstations, has an interface that is particularly well adapted to use in regular practice.

Integration in a Hospital Information System: HELP

The HELP system (Health Evaluation through Logical Processing), developed at the Latter Days Saints (LDS) Hospital in Salt Lake City, Utah, is a good example of a decision support system integrated into a hospital information system [Pryor 1987]. It operates in semi-active mode, and updating patient records triggers the decision support modules. A few examples illustrate how this integration works.

The warning system detects abnormal values of laboratory data or inadequate dosages. Diagnoses are proposed in some cases (problems in the acid–base equilibrium). For example, the model to track infectious diseases uses a knowledge base developed by specialists in the area. It analyzes microbiological data and compares it with other data available on the system (e.g., clinical results, patient files, surgery, pharmacy or radiology), signals the infections, and warns the pharmacists about administering antibiotics, the cost of treatment, or the length of time a drug should be administered. The system triggers a warning if it detects a nosocomial infection, an infection in a normally sterile site, an abnormal resistance, the use of an antibiotic that is too expensive, an overlong antibiotic treatment or an untreated or improperly treated infection. After installing the program, the number of cases of surgery patients receiving antibiotic treatment too late dropped from 27% to 14%, and the rate of postoperative infections dropped significantly from 1.9% to 0.9% [Evans 1985]. It also appears that in several cases patients received antibiotic treatments longer than their clinical state required.

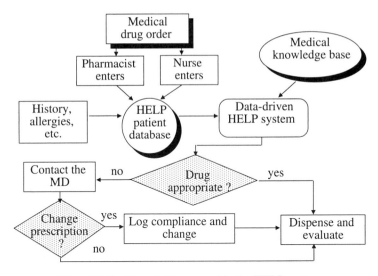

Figure 12.7 : Prescription control in the HELP system
(adapted from [Gardner 1990])

Figure 12.7 illustrates the organization of the system for controlling thera-peutic prescriptions. Prescriptions are entered interactively, and immediately controlled. Warnings are displayed if necessary. The hospital pharmacy committee, made up of physicians, pharmacists and pharmacologists, main-tains the knowledge base with the logical criteria for controlling prescrip-tions. Alerts are generated for allergies and interactions between drugs, between drugs and diets, drugs and dosages, drugs and diseases, and between the laboratory dosage and the drug dosage. For example, the system will sug-gest checking creatinine every 3 days if the patient is treated by an aminogly-coside. An evaluation carried out over a 12 month period showed that 8.45% of patients received warnings. This alert was vital for 49 patients (1.8%). Most physicians adhere strongly to the system's recommendations, and their numbers have increased steadily, from 71% in 1978 to 99% in 1988.

Each request for a blood product passes through the computer system, which checks the validity of the request in view of the patient's history and according to precise rules [Lepage 1991].

Decision Support in Molecular Biology

Genetic engineering techniques have developed over the past 20 years and have made the genes of simple and complex living organisms directly acces-sible for analysis. They have created a biological and medical revolution. In biology, they have made possible the understanding of the evolution of organisms and the adaptation of genomes to the environment. In the medical domain, they have enabled progress in understanding diseases, improving diagnoses for treatment and prevention.

This progress has been made possible by computers, which are used throughout the entire process of DNA analysis [Hunter 1993, Smith 1994]. For example:

- Gene sequencing is carried out by dividing genes into small segments of approximately 300 bases. Aligning multiple fragments manually would be impossible. Computer software helps in sequencing and limits the risk of error.

- Location of particular sequences is aided by the existence of computerized knowledge bases. Microbiology, for example, uses software to recognize bacteria by enzyme digestion after *polymerase chain reactions amplification* (PCR). These programs determine the enzymes or the combinations of enzymes that will generate restriction maps to differentiate several strains, using sequences from the strains to be isolated and break points of each one for the candidate enzymes.

- Comparing sequences obtained with known sequences requires access to various databases. The BISANCE system, developed in France, can compare a sequence to the NBRF (National Biomedical Research Foundation) protein bank and to two international nucleic acid banks, GenBank and EMBL (European Molecular Biology Laboratory). It is accessible via the Internet.

This chain requires the management of large databases storing tens of thousands of genome fragments that are updated constantly, and processing tools that use mathematical algorithms requiring enormous processing power.

Discussion and Conclusion

The usefulness and the limitations of decision support systems should be considered on several levels. We must analyze a system's functions, the type of consultation, its methodology, different factors concerning acceptance, such as the quality of the user interface, and the degree of integration in the information system.

In consultant systems, currently the most common, the physician decides if assistance is needed and, if so, must identify the most appropriate system. This type of consultation is not the easiest or the most efficient. Consultant systems must be integrated into larger information systems and tied to patient databases in order to play a more active role.

In applications that assist in the practice of medicine, it is not generally possible to separate diagnostic assistance from the medical procedures that identify a pathological state. It is not realistic today to create a system that would provide assistance in diagnosing a morbid state as accurately as possible. In practice, the process of refining a diagnosis stops when the therapeutic procedure is identical, whatever the results of the refinement. Instead, we must develop systems to help choose investigation strategies and to rationally propose additional examinations. These systems must be judged by the strategies they suggest and not by their diagnostic results.

On the methodological level, the difficulties in evaluating a decision support system should not be underestimated. Validation is a weighty, complex process for systems such as these. There are multiple evaluation criteria, often difficult to quantify, and evaluation bias is common. Vigorous validation procedures help evaluate a system's ability to meet its specifications.

The medical community's perception of decision support systems and the role they will play are two determining factors for the acceptance of these systems. Decision support systems must not be perceived as interfering with physicians' freedom in prescribing treatments, which is very important to them. In any case, making the appropriate decision is the physician's duty. Medical decision support systems should first be developed in areas where knowledge is clearly identified and generally agreed upon. This will prevent professionals from perceiving the advice as a constraint or a limitation on their activity.

Exercises

- *List and describe the main methods for medical decision support systems. Discuss their benefits, recommended usage, and limitations.*
- *Describe the major types of situations where medical decision support systems are used.*
- *Define and list the objectives of artificial intelligence in medicine.*
- *Define and list the objectives of a medical expert system.*
- *Describe the recommended use, feasibility, and limitations of expert systems.*
- *What are the main methods of reasoning used in decision support systems? Give some medical examples.*
- *Give some examples of expert systems useful in medicine and biology.*

13

Computer-Based Education

Introduction

The practice of medicine implies an aptitude for decision-making based on continuously updated knowledge. The extent of that knowledge can only increase. The goal of medical education is to prepare tomorrow's physicians by providing them with the knowledge required to practice medicine. It must also help students master the technologies necessary to manage and process medical information. These technologies are involved in the processes of building, communicating, and validating knowledge. Computer-based education (CBE) can be used by itself or as a complement to traditional methods. The large number of tools available represent situations that educators have identified and developed to assist in the learning process. Pedagogical materials related to a session must be structured and put in a form that can be used by educational software.

The Need for a Global Pedagogical Approach

Research on computer-based education and its developments has made practical and theoretical contributions to teaching. It uses epistemology, psychology, linguistics, and the cognitive sciences in general. It helps identify useful pedagogical techniques. The method analyzes and evaluates various teaching strategies to select and/or combine the most efficient ones.

The diagram developed by Harmon and King [Harmon 1985] (Figure 13.1) illustrates the two major types of knowledge: academic knowledge and knowledge gained from experience. The latter can be encouraged and amplified with appropriate pedagogical methods. To simplify, the form and goals of traditional education facilitate the acquisition of theories and general principles. Heuristic learning works better when based on practical experience and training, which is particularly useful in the actual practice of medicine.

In general, medical training is aimed at adults, whose pedagogical requirements are fundamentally different from those of children and adolescents. This population has the following characteristics:

- Adult students are self-motivated, while children tend to have a more passive attitude.
- Adults' intellectual organization is much more stable and less malleable than that of children. Someone teaching adults acts more as a stimulator than a trainer.
- Adults are the actors, not the audience. They are not trained; they train themselves. Adults may enjoy attending a conference given by an expert but tend to avoid formal lectures that duplicate theoretical teachings, which can be better presented in a book.
- Adults think in terms of usefulness for their work. They are not motivated by examinations, especially as they advance in their professional careers.

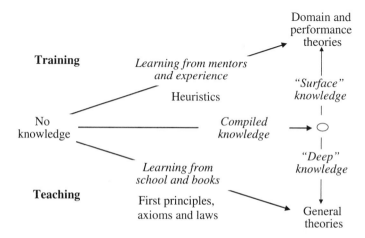

Figure 13.1 : Knowledge and education (adapted from [Harmon 1985])

On the one hand, we must facilitate the step between primary- and university-level education by encouraging young students to rapidly adopt an adult attitude towards education. On the other hand, once they have finished their schooling, physicians need assistance in adapting to the rapid changes in medical techniques and knowledge. Traditional medical training and the associated control of knowledge tend to overplay the importance of memorization. Students' efforts are oriented in this direction and they take on a passive role in acquiring knowledge. Although the length of studies has changed little, the volume and the content of programs increase constantly. Indeed, the learning and decision-making processes (how to access, acquire, and use knowledge to optimize medical decisions) do not receive enough attention. Most educational programs include classical initial training, but the rapid evolution of medical knowledge and practice requires continual training and ongoing validation of a physician's knowledge.

One of the major objectives in teaching medicine is *learning how to learn*. This approach requires pedagogical efforts in the following areas:

- Helping the learner (first a student, then a practicing physician) to define his or her individual objectives and training needs and then planning the required steps [Lemaitre 1989].
- Individualizing the relationship with the learner and adapting the teaching to each student's level.
- Increasing the quantity of individual work (e.g., updating knowledge, practical exercises, self-control).
- Increasing personal reflection (e.g., thinking about the educational process, critical study of decision-making situations, validating knowledge, etc.).

The Role of Computer-Based Education

In this context, the numerous CBE programs, or *courseware,* that have been developed show that it is possible to extend the range of pedagogical methods and to avoid some of the constraints of traditional education. CBE software presents the following theoretical advantages over traditional methods:

- Courseware provides greater autonomy to the student and can individualize the educational process. Students can learn at their own speed about the subjects that interest them or those they want to study further.
- Students learn interactively. Courseware lets users go back immediately for more information on any question or action and encourages their active participation.
- The recreational aspects of some courseware can motivate students to learn.
- The combination of various multimedia techniques facilitates memorization. Video sequences with spoken and written text, graphics, and images solicit different types of memory. Sequences can be repeated as often as necessary until learned.
- Computers let students simulate experimental situations that are not possible in a clinical environment or that may be dangerous to the patient (e.g., simulating surgical procedures).
- The learning process can be coupled with sequences to test a student's knowledge, so progress can be tested at any time. Errors can be corrected immediately without waiting for final examinations or actual medical practice.
- Some students are afraid to speak in public and even more afraid to make mistakes in front of their colleagues. They feel less inhibited with a computer.
- The use of courseware can be measured statistically and then improved or adapted accordingly.

Unfortunately courseware cannot simulate the complexity and subtlety of student–teacher, student–patient, or physician–patient relationships. Furthermore, a global and balanced education must include these tools while defining their role and establishing procedures to evaluate their actual pedagogical value.

Methods and Implementations

Courseware can contribute to the various phases of the pedagogical process: presenting information, repetition, control, and usage in simulations or in real situations.

Tutorial Training

The goal of tutorial training is to replace or complement traditional academic training provided in formal lectures and traditional educational materials (i.e., books, photocopies, films, etc.)

Programmed Training and Authoring Languages

In programmed training courseware, the information is divided into lessons that are presented in a certain order, as illustrated in Figure 13.2. Everything is planned ahead of time. Students are asked questions to test what they have learned. If the answer is correct, the lesson continues.

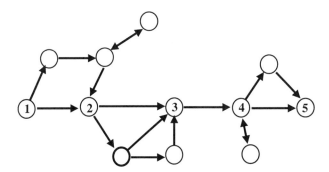

Figure 13.2 : Organization diagram of programmed teaching software

Specialized languages have been developed so that the author of the courseware does not have to learn traditional programming languages such as BASIC or Pascal, which are not suited to certain types of lessons. These are called *authoring languages*.

Numerous applications have been developed. They profit from the educators' experience and "encapsulate" it into programs that can reproduce it. The PLATO system (Programmed Logic for Automated Teaching Operations), developed at the University of Illinois at the end of the 1970s, is one of the most important systems in medicine. Based on a very complete authoring language, it has been used to create modules representing over 12,000 hours of courseware. More recent systems make extensive use of hypertext and hypermedia. Students are no longer obliged to follow an organization fixed by the professor or the rigid, linear structure of a book. Knowledge is accessible in a multitude of ways and can be presented in several forms, including graphics, images, and sounds. The ADAM® system developed for teaching anatomy is a significant example (figure 13.3).

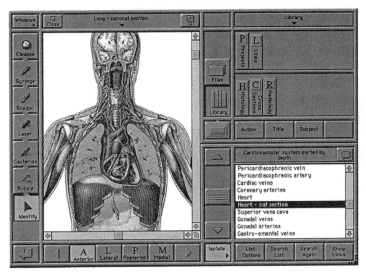

Figure 13.3 : A simple screen from the ADAM® teaching system (compliment of the ADAM corp.)

A growing amount of teaching material is currently rewritten in HTML format and made available via the Internet.

Tests show that the amount of knowledge acquired using these methods is at least equal to the knowledge obtained through traditional courses and that the time spent learning may be reduced.

Testing Knowledge

Procedures to test knowledge are part of teaching methods because questioning and repetition help to fix knowledge. Along with traditional editorial questions, several universities have adopted docimological methods that led to the development of knowledge evaluation systems based on questions with a limited number of answers. This simplified control process is well suited to computer processing. Question formats include true-false questions, multiple-choice questions, an ordered sequence of answers, and a "fill in the blank" answer to a text or graph. The pedagogical use of programs to manage test questions is limited, as are the benefits supplied by computers. They do provide useful aids in preparing examinations, particularly if a student's errors automatically generate reminders of the corresponding information. Their real value appears when they are coupled with programmed teaching methods that present and repeat information.

Modeling and Simulation

The practical use of anatomical or physiopathological knowledge can help students in acquiring useful problem-solving strategies in medicine. This may include making a diagnosis, prescribing a treatment, or following a patient's evolution over time. Simulations may be static or dynamic. In static simulations, students are presented with a predefined problem and must identify it. This problem does not change over the course of the simulation. In dynamic simulations, the patient's state evolves over time and according to the student's actions, thus providing a very useful training system.

Modeling and Simulating Biological Phenomena

Models of physiological processes can be very helpful in perceiving and understanding relationships between actions and their consequences. With known models, students can observe the results of changes in parameters and the evolution of the system. Simulations of the cardiovascular system, the physiology of respiration, or electrolytic disorders, for example, are extremely beneficial for understanding the complex processes involved. The graphic possibilities of modern technology are particularly useful.

Simulating Clinical Cases

Clinical simulations are used in diagnostic or therapeutic research to test students' clinical competence, to acquire heuristics for the generation of hypotheses, and to acquire experience in making diagnoses or deciding on treatments.

The CBX system (*computer-based examination*), developed by the *National Board of Medical Examiners* in the United States, is a good example of this type of application [Clyman 1990]. It simulates clinical situations and records the recommended actions as well as the student's response time. This information is later evaluated by a group of experts. Videodisks can be used to present various medical images (e.g., X-rays or pathology sections) as well as physiological signals.

The HeartLab program, developed on Apple Macintosh computers at Harvard Medical School, Boston, Massachusetts, teaches the basics of cardiac osculation and how to recognize the sounds of an abnormal heartbeat [Bergeron 1989]. Figure 13.4 represents a display from this system. By placing the stethoscope at different points on the diagram of the thorax displayed by the computer, the student hears sounds from these points according to the patient's position and the phase of breathing (inhaling or exhaling). This program is used in over one hundred medical schools in the United States.

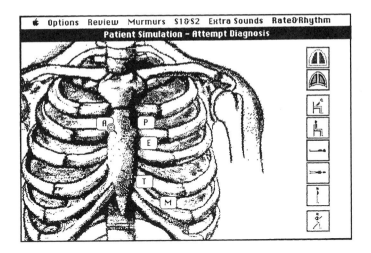

Figure 13.4 : A case simulation screen from HeartLab (courtesy of de B. Bergeron and colleagues, Harvard Medical School, Boston, Massachusetts)

The TIME project, developed at the National Library of Medicine in Bethesda, Maryland, is based on simulations of patient cases recorded on videodisk [Harless 1986]. Each disk contains various scenes showing the patient in the hospital and his clinical history (using flashback techniques from the cinema), clinical examinations, or test results. Scenes are presented upon student request. The students can interrogate patients using a voice recognition system, ask for additional tests or X-rays, and visualize the results. The simulation is very realistic and provides immediate reactions. The patient's condition will improve or decline according to the student's decisions. The intensive use of multimedia technologies such as videodisks, voice recognition, sound, and touch screens makes the system attractive to users. Simulated medical emergencies are realistic, credible, and require real-time decisions.

The ILIAD system, developed on Apple Macintosh systems at the University of Utah, Salt Lake City, simulates cases for internal medicine [Warner 1988, Cundick 1989, Bouhaddou 1995]. Its strategy is based on the *a priori* probabilities of the various diseases, the predictive value of the signs observed, and the cost of tests that have been proposed or performed.

On-Site Teaching

This approach attempts to provide access to training and decision support systems during visits at the bedside or the doctor's office. These intelligent assistants are designed to advise the physician on a given clinical situation. They have a stronger pedagogical impact than specialized tools designed for teaching, while helping to improve the quality of health care. The psychological involvement of the physician in training, who wants to provide the best possible care to the patient, is an important motivational factor in training and learning. Training becomes a focused, ongoing activity.

Initially, the system may be limited to facilitating access to specialized knowledge. Systems for managing health-care units or hospital information systems such as HELP (which provides access to information bases or knowledge bases concerning tests, procedures, therapy, etc.) have demonstrated the usefulness of providing contextual knowledge at the right place and at the right time. This automatic "knowledge coupling" encourages physicians to improve the physician–patient relationship and to keep reliable medical records, on the one hand, and to trust the computer for access to book knowledge on the other hand [Weed 1991].

Integrating pedagogical decision support systems in clinical management systems is more ambitious as the integrated system can directly participate in the student's decisions. The creation of "critical" expert systems, able to analyze and discuss the accuracy of users' proposals, provides a complement to traditional decision-making methods.

Intelligent CBE Systems

The borderlines between tutorial systems, clinical simulation tools, and decision support tools used for training are not immovable. The normal educational model used for most CBE applications uses cybernetic commands and controls. If we consider education as a "process of communication and cooperation", this paradigm must be reconsidered, and the limitations of traditional CBE become apparent. Traditional tutorial systems are not very adaptable and do not systematically respond to students' reactions. Educational software should be based on more complex cognitive models and follow a pedagogical strategy helping the student to take the initiative related to his or her level of knowledge.

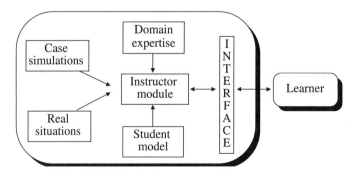

Figure 13.5 : General architecture of an intelligent computer-based
education system (ICBE)

The GUIDON NEOMYCIN system, developed at Stanford University, California, is one of the first prototypes of an intelligent CBE system [Clancey 1986, 1987]. It uses the knowledge base of the MYCIN expert system (see Chapter 4) and its own strategic rules to teach diagnostic and therapeutic rules for meningitis.

Figure 13.5 presents a simplified diagram of the architecture for an intelligent computer-based education (ICBE) system. The training module's intelligence evaluates the student's reasoning, based on its knowledge of the field, and guides the student using an adapted teaching strategy. The student communicates with the CBE system using a friendly, well-adapted interface. The explanations are adapted to the student's level.

The system diagnoses the student's errors, improving the system's pertinence and efficiency. The goal is to help the student exploit the necessary knowledge and ignore the irrelevant one. Figure 13.6 shows an example of a model for diagnosing errors based on the knowledge used in decision-making.

What is currently done:	Take into account correct knowledge and nonpertinent knowledge		Errors due to bias	Errors due to lack of experience
	Nonpertinent knowledge	**Correct knowledge**	**Knowledge not taken into account**	**Missing knowledge**
What should be done:	Ignore nonpertinent knowledge	Use the necessary knowledge		

Figure 13.6 : Diagnosis of errors and knowledge involved in a decision (adapted from [Silvermann 1991])

Discussion and Conclusion

Data processing technologies are a major asset for improving the quality of medical training. Microcomputers have significantly contributed to the spread of CBE by directly or indirectly bringing information to the physician's desktop through communication networks. Hypertext techniques and hypermedia systems make learning easier by stimulating different memorization systems in the brain (visual, auditory) and encouraging interaction with the computer. Interactive videodisks can place the student in more realistic situations than previous technologies. Artificial intelligence has shown the importance of an approach based on the structure of knowledge. It can help students understand the complexity and multiplicity of reasoning mechanisms and better separates what computers can do from what they cannot.

Models of the expert, the tutor, and the student can be integrated in CBE tools to make them more useful and better adapted.

These technological perspectives should not lead to overly optimistic conclusions. Several barriers are present when developing any training program (with or without computers):

- Knowledge transfer is a slow process, requiring significant human resources.
- Professors, whose careers depend mainly on their research, are not inclined to develop pedagogical tools.
- People are not always ready to share pedagogical materials. Even if these were shared, there are currently no standard educational software development tools that can group components into larger constructs.
- Medical schools do not always have appropriate or sufficient computer equipment. Ideally, each student should have his or her own computer at home.

The benefits of CBE techniques must also be studied and quantified more methodically. We must evaluate existing systems and their pedagogical possibilities, which should not be confused with user satisfaction. The rare studies that do exist tend to prove that students can learn faster (between 30% and 50%) and better retain what they learned through CBE. The decreasing cost of computers and the development of multimedia systems and communication networks should help to overcome current limitations in distributing and updating these systems.

Exercises

- *List the advantages and disadvantages of CBE compared to traditional methods.*
- *Identify the various types of CBE systems and discuss their place in an overall educational system.*
- *List some of the major barriers to developing CBE systems.*

14

Analysis and Control of Medical Activity

Introduction

The cost of health care continues to rise in most countries. Several factors are responsible for this phenomenon: the development of new medical techniques, the increased scope of health care, the aging of the population, improvements in the standard of living, and a general population that is better informed about needs and demand. In parallel, the use of inappropriate therapeutic techniques and unproductive or dangerous investigatory techniques is difficult to control and can cause major discrepancies in medical practice. Increased costs are not synonymous with increased health-care quality, and reorganizing the health-care system does not guarantee improvement in the quality of health care provided.

This situation calls for some regulatory mechanism and an optimal distribution of resources as well as the selection of criteria that help to reconcile the practice of quality medicine, required by medical ethics, and economic necessities.

This chapter provides a few definitions and general principles that may be helpful in the quantitative and qualitative evaluation of health care.

Controlling Health-Care Expenses

Administrative data alone do not provide the complete picture of medical activity required for controlling health-care expenses and maintaining or improving the quality of the care provided to the entire population. This control requires a thorough knowledge of the process of cost production in health care, directly linked to the type of medical problems to be solved, and the results obtained, which must be related to the medical decisions made. It requires very detailed knowledge of the initial situation and a well-researched estimate of health needs and goals. To understand the costs involved, we must relate them to the pathologies treated as well as the results obtained in terms of the patient's state of health or quality of life.

The reform of French hospitals in 1983 (Act of August 11, 1983) introduced "global endowment", determined essentially by the level of operating expenses expected for the year. As a result, the indicators used by hospitals and the methods used to calculate expenses are critical during budget negotiations with supervising bodies. In order to improve the activity indicators, the French administration for hospitals (*Directic.. des Hôpitaux*) introduced at the same period a national program for "medicalizing" computer systems, known as PMSI (for *Programme de Médicalisation du Système d'Informa-tion*). In its : ˙ al phase, this system was based on the *diagnosis related groups* (DRG) approach developed by Fetter and colleagues at Yale univer-sιʋ, New Haven, Connecticut, for describing hospital production [Fetter 1980, Frutiger 1991]. It will have to be completed by quality measurements.

Federal evaluation policy in the United States led to an approach entitled *evidence-based medicine* that defines guidelines and quality controls (illustrated in Figure 14.1). It is used by two federal agencies: the Agency for Health Care Policy and Research (AHCPR) and the Health Care Financing Administration (HCFA). *Clinical Practice Guidelines* are developed by committees of experts. These guidelines are taught in medical schools to improve health-care quality and used to evaluate how medical practice conforms to the guidelines as well as the results obtained. New rules are then established to improve quality.Conformity with quality assurance programs is validated by the Joint Commission on the Accreditation of Hospital Organizations (JCAHO).

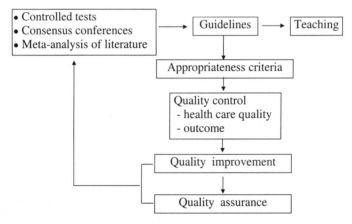

Figure 14.1 : The evidence-based medicine approach

Evaluation, Control, and Quality

The word *evaluation* has several definitions and covers a large number of applications. Administrators, economists, and physicians use the term to mean different things, often leading to misinterpretations and confusion. Furthermore, the scope of evaluations is large and the concept is often confused with control or quality.

	Evaluation	**Control**
Objective	Search for non-quality	Search for abuses and fraud
References	Medical recommendations	Regulations: • Administrative • Medical references
Scope	Representative sample of professionals	Professionals identified by measuring activity
Principle	Honesty does not guarantee performance	Suspicion of fraud and abuse
Measure-ments	• Respecting procedures and instructions • Patient satisfaction • Costs of non-quality	How well activities conform to medical and administrative regulations (invoicing, nomenclatures, conventions)
Actions	In case of non-quality: • Systematic actions: - Training - Organization of treatment • Behavioral action (for health-care providers, patients, and the population)	In case of infringement: • Penalties • Legal action

Figure 14.2 : Differences between health-care evaluation and control
(adapted from [Béraud 1995])

Figures 14.2 and 14.3, based on the work of C. Béraud [Béraud 1995], summarize the characteristics of these concepts based on their objectives, their references, scope of action, personnel involved, and challenges:

	Evaluating medical practice	**Health-care quality**
Objective	Correct	Prevent
Activity	Temporary	Permanent
Personnel	Physicians	All
Target	Punctual	Global
Stakes	Defining and developing health-care procedures	Organizing health-care procedures

Figure 14.3 : Evaluating medical practice and health-care quality
(adapted from [Béraud 1995])

"The evaluation of medical practice, in the form of a detailed medical audit, reveals non-quality by measuring the difference between practice and medical recommendations. Quality is an objective that helps avoid non-quality. Quality is not corrected but built, and, once built, it can be guaranteed through quality assurance." [Béraud 1995]

Methods and Principles for Analyzing Medical Activity

A General Model

Medico-economic analyses of medical activities model medical interventions. Figure 14.4 illustrates the problem in a hospital environment. A hospital is considered as a set of resources for producing health care. The results should be an improvement of patients' overall state of health. Various indicators help to evaluate operations:

- *Efficiency* can be analyzed by comparing the resources used (input into the health-care system), expressed in terms of material, human, and administrative resources, and the activity (output of the system), expressed in terms of medical treatment performed (consultation, hospitalizations, examinations, etc.).
- *Effectiveness* relates the activity and its product, expressed in terms of medical problems solved (medical diagnostics, homogeneous groups of patients, case mix, etc.).
- *Resource utilization* correlates resources with activity or production.
- *Quality assessment* relates the hospital's activity or production with the results of the activity or production. Did an examination lead to the correct diagnosis? Did the treatment improve the patient's health?

This general model may be adapted to various health-care structures (public or private hospitals, doctor's offices, preventive medical centers, etc.).

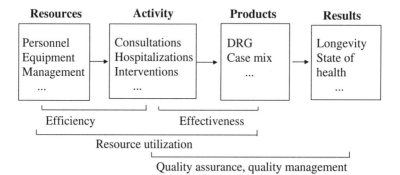

Figure 14.4 : General model of medical-economic evaluation

Evaluating Costs

Several concepts are involved when calculating production costs and expenses:

- A *product* is a good or a service, usually one that is sold. In the health arena, care provided for a medical or surgical problem is the product.
- *Structural* or *fixed costs* are related to the company's existence.
- *Operating expenses*, or variable expenses, are related to production volumes.
- *Direct costs* are incurred when providing services (material, personnel, operations). They include committed costs and operating expenses.
- *Indirect costs* cannot be directly attributed to services provided but require intermediate calculations (e.g., administrative expenses).
- *Marginal costs* are defined as the increase of overall costs related to the production of an additional unit. We can calculate the marginal cost of an additional diagnostic case or an additional X-ray examination to be performed.
- The *average cost* is the total cost divided by the number of service units produced.

Three types of analyses are generally used for economic evaluations:

- *Cost–benefit analyses* compare two (or more) procedures by evaluating their costs and their results expressed in monetary units. They require users to put a cost on human life (the estimation of gains and losses related to prolonging life or a state of health). They attempt to answer the question: Is the purpose of the procedure acceptable?
- *Cost–efficiency analyses* compare two (or several) procedures by evaluating their costs in monetary units (dollars) and their results in physical units (the number of years life is extended or diseases are avoided). These analyses attempt to evaluate the efficiency of an operation designed to reach a specific goal.
- *Cost–utility analyses* compare two (or several) procedures by evaluating their costs in monetary units and their results expressed qualitatively, such as improvement in the quality of life.

The concepts of costs and benefits are particularly difficult to define for new technologies whose implications cover the short, medium, and long term and involve several categories of players. For example, although the benefits of a hospital information system may be obvious, they are difficult to isolate and quantify. Productivity gains may lead to the implementation of the system as a set of procedures related to the hospital's restructuring.

Two Approaches for "Medicalized" Management

Normalized Approach

Starting with the analysis of clearly defined medical situations, this method attempts to determine the criteria for "proper treatment" and publishes these criteria as standards. It assumes that such standards can be practically determined and widely distributed in the medical community. The consensus conference approach is based on this method.

Explanatory Approach

Starting with the analysis of medical-economic data, this approach searches for statistical links between the various factors, suggests causal links, and eventually proposes strategies for treatment. It includes the following steps:

- Defining the factors to be explained (dependent variables) such as the duration or the cost of hospitalization;
- Identifying explanatory factors (independent variables) such as the main medical diagnosis and secondary diagnoses, the severity of the case, age, gender, surgical procedures, and the patient's progress at the end of the stay;
- Using statistical methods to evaluate the explanatory capabilities of the independent variables;
- Comparing procedures to the average and analyzing the deviations;
- Eventually making suggestions for new explanatory hypotheses;
- Making suggestions for procedural strategies.

The explanatory method presumes that statistical analysis can define procedural profiles and can analyze any deviation from a mean behavior.

Analyzing Medical Activity in the Hospital

Resource Indicators

Resources concern personnel (their number and qualifications), materials (type and technical capabilities), and organizational structures (administrative and technical services). In France, hospital structures are organized into a hierarchy of services or responsibility centers (RC) that may be grouped into departments. A responsibility center may be subdivided into activity centers (AC), which in turn may be divided into functional units (FU), the smallest medical-administrative entity in the hospital. Each functional unit is assigned human resources, technical resources (e.g., intensive-care or X-ray equipment), or hospital beds.

Activity Indicators

Overall activity may be expressed as a number of admissions, hospital stays (short, medium, and long stays), the number of days hospitalized, the number of consultations, or the number of medical procedures performed. Encoding diagnoses and procedures often causes problems because the nomenclatures are not well adapted (see Chapter 5).

Based on these activity indicators and resource indicators, we can calculate overall resource usage indicators. They mainly concern:

- the average length of hospitalization and patient distribution and

- the utilization of resources and structures such as work load, bed occupancy rates, consulting facilities or examination equipment.

Production Indicators

Production indicators evaluate the hospital's activity by measuring the diagnostic care provided without evaluating the results in terms of patients' health (i.e., the efficiency and utility of the procedures).

Homogenous Patient Groups

Homogenous patient groups (Groupes Homogènes de Malades or GHM) are an adaptation of the U.S. system of Diagnosis Related Groups (DRG), developed by the team led by R. Fetter at Yale University [Fetter 1990]. In this model, a hospital's product is defined by groups of hospitalizations presenting relative clinical similarities and using similar resources. This description cannot present hospital activity in terms of the quality of health care provided. Its empirical construction was guided by the following requirements:

- The classification had to be functional. The number of homogenous groups created was limited to provide a useful tool: 470 groups were defined.
- The amount of information describing each patient hospitalized was limited (10 to 15 data elements) to allow routine, exhaustive data collection in all hospital services. Furthermore, information had to be easily obtained, unambiguous, and reliable.
- Each group had to be clinically coherent. The grouping system was verified by clinical technicians.
- Each group had to contain patients that used the same type of resources.
- The length of hospitalization was selected as an approximate measure of resource usage because it was simple and readily available.
- The system had to be interactive so that clinical technicians could participate in its development. The result is not a simple statistical classification.

The DRGs were developed interactively using the automatic interaction detector (AID) program. The classification algorithm created groups whose variations, calculated on the selected dependent variable, had the two following properties:

- the lowest possible variation within each group and
- the greatest possible variation between groups.

For each hospitalization to be classified, defined by independent variables, the algorithm identifies the variables that explain as much of the variation as possible in order to create groups that meet the two criteria above. This operation is reiterated to create new partitions. At each step, the pertinence of the groups created is clinically judged by experts. These experts either used the proposed division or create a division manually using non-statistical criteria to make groups more medically homogenous.

	Categories	Surgery	Medicine	Total
1	Disorders of the nervous system	8	26	34
2	Disorders of the eye	7	6	13
3	Disorders of the ears, nose, throat, mouth, and teeth	17	14	31
4	Respiratory disorders	3	25	28
5	Disorders of the circulatory system	18	25	43
6	Disorders of the digestive tract	24	16	40
7	Disorders of the hepatobiliary system and pancreas	11	7	18
8	Disorders and trauma of the musculoskeletal system and connective tissue	27	22	49
9	Cutaneous, subcutaneous, and breast-related disorders	14	14	28
10	Endocrine, metabolic, and nutritional disorders	9	8	17
11	Disorders of the kidneys and the urinary tract	12	18	30
12	Male genital disorders	12	7	19
13	Female genital disorders	13	4	17
14	Pathological pregnancies, deliveries, and postnatal disorders	5	10	15
15	Disorders in newborns, premature babies, and during the prenatal period	0	7	7
16	Disorders of the blood or the hematopoetic system	3	5	8
17	Myeloproliferative disorders and tumors whose locations are unknown or generalized	6	9	15
18	Infectious diseases and parasitic diseases	1	8	9
19	Mental disorders	1	8	9
20	Drug-related or drug-induced organic mental problems	0	5	5
21	Trauma, allergies, and poisoning	5	12	17
22	Burns	2	3	5
23	Factors influencing the state of health and other reasons for using health services	1	6	7
24	Sessions and hospitalizations under 24 hours	22	29	51
	Total	**221**	**294**	**515**

Figure 14.5 : The major diagnostic categories and their French GHM numbers

The DRG classification used in France has some minor differences with the American system (Figure 14.5). Figure 14.6 presents a general overview of how the classification is organized and Figure 14.7 provides a simplified example of segmentation criteria used to build DRGs.

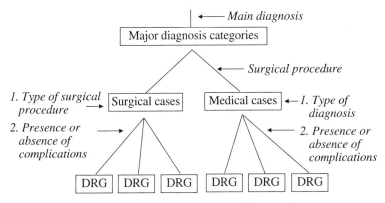

Figure 14.6 : The principle of DRG classifications

				DRG
Major procedures on the liver, the pancreas and the portal and venacaval veins				# 267
Minor procedures on the liver, the pancreas and the portal and venacaval veins				# 268
Procedures on the Biliary Tree (B.T.)	Total cholecystectomies	with exploration of the B.T.	Age > 69 and/or W.R.C.	# 271
			Age < 70 without R.C.	# 272
		without exploration of the B.T.	Age > 69 and/or W.R.C.	# 273
			Age < 70 without R.C.	# 274
	Other than total cholecystectomies	Age > 69 years and/or W.R.C.		# 269
		Age < 70 years without R.C.		# 270
Diagnostic surgery on the hepato-biliary system and the pancreas		For malignant diseases		# 275
		For benign diseases		# 276
Other procedures on the hepatobiliary and pancreatic systems				# 277

Figure 14.7 : Examples of French DRGs concerning disorders in the hepatobiliary system and the pancreas. W.R.C.: with related complications

Case Mix

The division of diseases into groups creates a case mix. This mix provides a rough estimation of hospital activity, as there is often considerable diversity in the medical classes within a single DRG. The effects of this grouping tend to mask the diversity of cases within one hospital or a group of hospitals.

Severity Index

These observations led to the development of complementary techniques to better represent the clinical situation and in particular the severity of cases.

- The *computerized severity index* (CSI), developed by Suzan Horn, relies on both ICD-9-CM diagnosis codes and key clinical findings. It begins with the patient's principal diagnosis and uses physiological markers to adjust the diagnosis. A score from 1 to 4 is assigned after consulting the medical records for each considered disease [Horn 1983, 1991].

- *Disease staging* (DS), developed by Joseph Gonella, bases the concept of risk on the probability of death due to complications for the declared diagnosis. A score from 1 to 4 is established by searching the medical records for signs of severity. Its major weakness is its purely clinical encoding system, which does not account for the resources used for treatment [Gonella 1984, Calore 1987].

- The Medis II groups (*Medical Illness Severity Grouping System* II), developed by the Mediqual company, base the concept of risk on the probability of the failure of a vital organ. A score is calculated 48 hours after hospitalization and then again after 5 days by searching the medical records for predetermined and validated key clinical findings [Brewster 1985].

- *Patient Management Categories* (PMCs), mainly based on a statistical approach, are an alternative to DRGs. The 840 classes are based on determining the clinical paths used according to the diagnostic and/or clinical procedures used during the hospitalization [Young 1982, 1994].

- The most recent version of DRG, called RDRG (*Refined DRG*), developed by the team at Yale, improves the system's ability to consider case severity. In particular, it identifies special associations between primary and secondary diagnoses. This is a group of diagnoses that become critical for assigning a case to a particular DRG [Freeman 1995].

- The APACHE III score is widely used in intensive care. It can classify diseases according to their severity 24 hours after admission [Knaus 1985, 1991].

Method	CSI	DS	Medis	PMCs
Method of gathering data	Clinical data-based	Discharge abstract-based	Clinical data-based	Discharge abstract-based
Data used	Diagnostic and disease-specific variables	Diagnostic codes	Over 250 key clinical findings	Diagnostic codes
Number of disease groups	800	400	67	840
Type of score	Ordinal 0 to 4	Ordinal 1 to 4	Ordinal 0 to 4	Interval
Probability of in-hospital death		yes	yes	

Figure 14.8 : Examples of severity measures for comparing hospital death rates (adapted from [Aronow 1988, Iezzoni 1997])

Figure 14.8 presents some of the characteristics of four of these systems for evaluating severity [Aronow 1988, Iezzoni 1997]. Several methods consider precise physiological or medical problems without taking into account the importance of accompanying chronic diseases or the patient's problem as a whole. None of the current generation of severity measurement systems does provide a totally satisfactory solution [Iezzoni 1997].

The French System for Processing Hospitalization Reports

The goal of the French program for "medicalizing" information systems (PMSI for *Programme de Médicalisation du Système d'Information*) is to standardize the way information is gathered for the standard discharge summary (*Résumé standardisé de sortie* or RSS) (Figure 14.9) for each patient hospitalized. It provides a DRG classification and an analysis of the hospital's case mix.

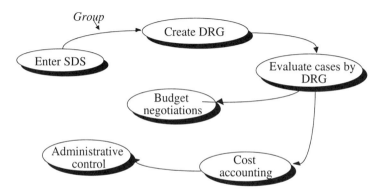

Figure 14.9 : Steps for installing the French PMSI program

The descriptive variables of the hospitalization concern four entities: the patient, the disease, the medical treatment, and the health-care structure. This information is gathered by each medical unit to create the medical unit discharge summary (*résumé d'unité médicale* or RUM). The RSS is a series of RUMs, each of which uses the format described in Figure 14.10. This series of RUMs covers the entire hospitalization.

A medical unit is defined as a functional unit, a service (responsibility center), or an activity center (group of functional units). Primary and secondary diagnoses are encoded using the international classification of diseases published by the WHO (10th revision). To encode procedures, the French Health Ministry established a codification by type of procedure (see Chapter 8). Sessions (see category 24 of figure 14.5) concern iterative care (e.g., dialysis, chemotherapy, etc.).

Two main organizations have been tested for gathering the information for RSSs:

1	Hospital ID number
2	RUM format version
3	RUM number
4	Date of birth
5	Sex
6	Medical unit number
7	Date entered in the unit
8	Mode entered in the unit
9	Origin (if change or transfer)
10	Date left unit
11	Mode left unit
12	Destination (if change or transfer)
13	Total hospitalization less than 24 hours
14	Hospitalized in the previous 30 days
15	Home postal code
16	Weight at birth (for newborns)
17	Number of sessions
18	Main diagnosis
19	Number of associated diagnostics (d) in this RUM
20	Number of procedures (p) in this RUM
21	Reserved
22	Associated diagnostics (1 to d)
23	Procedures (1 to p)

Figure 14.10 : Information in a medical unit discharge summary (RUM

- centralized RSS encoding, where a group of specially trained employees encode patient records in a central location, and enter this information into the computer; and

- decentralized encoding, where the medical services encode the information themselves with the active participation of practitioners.

The second method seems preferable. To establish a useful and efficient computer system, the information produced by a service should be processed by that service. Having practitioners encode their own activities encourages dialogue that prepares for a pertinent analysis and a better understanding of the results. On the other extreme, centralized encoding places the evaluation process outside the service's activities. Encoding in highly specialized areas is best performed by experts.

In theory, centralized encoding provides more regular encoding, but this advantage is overestimated. It ignores the fact that there cannot be a consensus among experts on a given medical problem and neglects the difficulties experts have in defining clear rules for encoding that ensure true regularity. Furthermore, the daily practice of medicine presents problems that are difficult to describe. For example, a patient presents lithiasis of the biliary tree and acute pancreatic problems. This may be described as cholelithiasis with pancreatic complications, or acute pancreatis caused by an impacted gallstone. The encoding is different for the two cases, and only the practitioner is able to select the one that best describes the situation.

After entering the RSSs, software programs divide the hospitalizations into homogenous patient groups and print statistics. The DRGs are clinically and statistically analyzed. The distribution of the length of hospital stays can be calculated for each DRG. This isolates the subgroups where the length of hospitalization varies dramatically within a DRG, and helps determine the medical (or organizational) reasons for these differences. In general, DRG analysis should help compare the activities of different hospitals given their own case mixes.

Quality Indicators

The economic dimension of medical information systems must be balanced by an emphasis on quality medicine that meets ethical criteria. Several steps are necessary for establishing a control and quality assurance system:

- Defining quality objectives.
- Identifying areas to be evaluated.
- Defining the factors to study and the indicators.
- Implementing procedures for gathering data and processing the results.
- Defining thresholds for intervention and actions to be taken.
- Verifying the efficiency of measures implemented and the maintenance of benefits observed.
- Communicating and distributing the results.

Quality of care can be defined as "the degree to which health services for individuals and populations increase the likelihood of desired health outcomes and are consistent with current professional knowledge" [Lohr 1990]. Quality objectives must therefore take into account the various players involved (patients, physicians, health-care personnel, administrators, etc.). The quality objectives set forth by the American Medical Association presented in Figure 14.11 are an example.

---

1) Provide optimal improvement in the patient's health
2) Promote better health and disease prevention
3) Work when required, i.e., at any time
4) Strive for informed patient cooperation and participation in the health-care and decision-making processes
5) Base activities on accepted principles of medical science
6) Keep the patient's interest in mind
7) Use technology efficiently
8) Remain sufficiently well-informed to provide continuous health-care and evaluate options
9) Take the patient's goals and values into account

Figure 14.11 : Quality objectives of the American Medical Association

There are several quality indicators, and they are closely related to the area being evaluated. These may be "positive" health indicators (e.g., improvement of the state of health, the quality of life, preventing complications, preventing drug side-effects, etc.) or the suppression of the effects or consequence of pathologies (e.g., correcting a risk factor, reducing a handicap, treating a debilitating disorder). Indicators should be as objective as possible. This may be relatively simple for a quantitative parameter such as the blood pressure or glycemia or much more difficult for subjective parameters such as well-being.

Discussion and Conclusion

The measurement and analysis of medical activity may be developed from an information processing chain that accounts for resources, activity, products, and results. The evaluation, essentially based on economic criteria, should be considered as a guide for judgment, not as a substitute. If quality is not built into the evaluation procedures, the health system will deteriorate, guided only by economic criteria that may contradict medical ethics. Furthermore, those commissioning and carrying out research must pay close attention to the conditions and the use of the chosen indicators, as suggested by Berwick [Berwick 1989]. Continuous data-gathering systems, based on quality objectives and providing ongoing quality control, provide greater motivation to the health-care team and in some cases are more useful than looking for deviations from average medical practice calculated on heterogeneous samples.

Multidisciplinary teams must be created to provide credible and acceptable results for any evaluation study. Economists, methodologists, and specialists must be involved for the results to impact and influence future choices and practice.

Exercises

- *Define the concepts of evaluation, control and quality of health care.*
- *What are the major areas of health-care evaluation?*
- *What is the principle of health-care guidelines? What should they provide?*
- *Explain the difference between utility, effectiveness, and efficiency, and give examples.*
- *Define the major types of costs.*
- *Explain the principle of diagnosis related groups (DRG), and discuss their limitations.*
- *Explain the principle of evaluating hospital activities by case mix.*
- *Discuss the principles and implementation of standard diagnostic summaries.*
- *Give some examples of indicators of health-care quality.*

15

Security and Data Protection

Introduction

Data processing technologies have created new risks concerning the privacy and protection of medical data. The development of computer networks, for example, while facilitating communication between players in the health-care system, also increases the danger of illicit access to confidential data. Poor quality of transmitted images in telemedicine may cause incorrect interpretations and diagnoses. These risks call for appropriate technical and organizational measures, especially when dealing with patients' medical records.

Identifying the Risks

Collecting, storing, and consulting information on computers offers possibilities that go beyond traditional paper-based records. It is much easier to access individual or collective information. This access can be medically unjustified or even malicious. Intrinsic risks are involved when using machines and media for memorizing data. Although failures are increasingly rare, they remain possible. Information may be lost, or records may be created with incorrect data, leading to poor medical decisions. The risks involving machines, data, and programs are numerous:

- Illegal access to computing centers;
- Equipment theft, made easier by miniaturization (microcomputers);
- Malicious use of data communication resources. This risk increases with the installation of networks like the Internet (see Chapter 1);
- Unauthorized modification of programs;
- Illegal consultation (with or without copying) of data. This risk increases with the use of microcomputers as workstations;
- Unauthorized or incorrect use of programs or functions;
- Hardware failures;
- Programming errors, especially when changing versions;
- Failures that occur when data is being updated;

- Attributing one patient's data to another person (improper identification, homonyms, etc.).

The diagram in Figure 15.1 illustrates these risks.

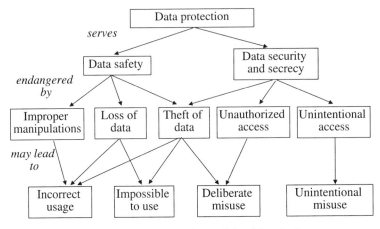

Figure 15.1 : Data protection and the risks of misuse
(adapted from [Griesser 1977])

Protecting Data Concerning Individuals

Data protection involves two aspects: integrity and security (Figure 15.1).

- *Integrity* means that data must be valid and accessible at all times. Data integrity may be affected by improper manipulation, but also by accidental or malicious loss of data. Computer viruses, the destruction of storage media, and other forms of computer sabotage are real problems for the integrity of patient databases.

- *Security* means data must be protected against unauthorized access (intentional or unintentional) contrary to the patient's interest, and that their privacy should be respected.

Professional Ethics and Legal Measures

The problems involved in computerizing medical data have been under close scrutiny in the past few years. Even if the ethical basis is nearly identical worldwide, the legal measures may vary widely between countries.

The International Principles

The World Medical Association [WMA 1985] has a very open position: it recognizes the advantages offered by computers in health and makes recommendations for broadly regulating the use of medical data to legitimate ends.

The International Conference Of Medical Professionals [CIOM 1987] has adopted a similar attitude in its principles used to create new codes of medical ethics. These international organizations state general principles and leave it up to the national professional medical organizations to apply them.

Article 6 of the Convention of the European Council dated January 28, 1981 stipulates that "data of a personal nature concerning health or sexual activities may not be processed automatically unless internal laws provide appropriate guarantees." This convention became effective in November, 1985. It requires all member countries to offer legal protection of sensitive medical data.

The Directive of the European Parliament and Council of October 24, 1995, extends the 1981 Convention and represents a further step towards the harmonization of European legislations.

The Situation in France

Different texts cover the problems of professional, medical, and data secrecy. They specify the patient's rights, his means of defense, and in general the regulations for protecting individual data.

Professional Secrecy

Professional secrecy is regulated by the professional code of medical ethics (*Code de Déontologie Médicale*) [CDM 1995], the public health code (*Code de la Santé Publique*) [CSP 1995], the law on data processing, data files, and individual liberties (*Loi informatique, fichiers et libertés*) [IFL 1978], and breaches of that confidence are covered by the penal code (*Code Pénal*) [CP 1995].

The code of medical ethics specifies that "Professional secrecy, created in the patients' interest, is required of all physicians as established by the law. This secrecy covers everything the physician learns when performing his duties, that is, everything he has been told, but also what he has seen, heard and understood" [CDM 1995, art. 4]. The code also specifies "the physician must make sure to protect against any indiscretion of his clinical records and documents that he may possess concerning his patients. When he uses them for scientific publication of his medical observations, he must make sure that patients cannot be identified" [CDM 1995, art. 73]. This respect of privacy covers all health professionals, pharmacists, nursing personnel, secretaries, and computer technicians who may access personal data.

Any negligence in respecting this confidence may be severely punished. Article 226-13 of the penal code stipulates: "Any person having knowledge of secrets by state or by profession or by permanent or temporary functions who reveals these secrets shall be punished by one year in prison and a fine of 100,000 French francs" [CP 1995, art. 226-13].

Law on "Computers, Files, and Freedom"

Most western countries have adopted legislation concerning the principles of protecting personal data. In France, the act of January 6, 1978, entitled "Data Processing, Data Files and Individual Liberties" (*Loi informatique, fichiers et libertés*), protects personal information and defines patients' rights (full text is available via the Internet at http://info.in2p3.fr/secur/legal/178-17-text.html) [IFL 1978]. It includes general measures concerning the development, use, and protection of computer files. The law was modified in July, 1994. It should be integrated with the existing articles of the code of medical ethics [CDM 1979, art. 11, 12, 13 and 42], the articles of the penal code concerning breaches of professional secrecy [CP, art. 226-13], the recommendations of the European Council of January 3, 1981 [CE 1981] and the directive of October 24, 1995, of the European Parliament and Council [EP 1995].

The first article of the law of January 6, 1978 states that "Data processing shall be at the service of every citizen. It shall develop in the context of international co-operation. It shall infringe neither human identity, nor the rights of man, nor privacy, nor individual or public liberties." [IFL 1978, art. 1].

This law states that individuals should be informed of any computer files containing personal information concerning them, and that the file cannot be created without their express consent. Furthermore, individuals have the right to access information concerning them. They may oppose such records and request any corrections they deem necessary [IFL 1978, art. 22, 26,34-40,45]. For medical data, this right is exercised by a physician designated by the patient.

The national commission on computers and liberties (*Commission Nationale de l'Informatique et des Libertés* or CNIL), an independent administrative body, is responsible for ensuring the law is correctly applied. It controls the formalities required of anyone who wants to process personal data on a computer. It can also carry out checks, controls, and warnings, and can denounce any infringements of the law.

Declaring Files Containing Personal Information

Any file containing personal data (medical or otherwise) must be declared to the CNIL. Personal information means data that describes a clearly identified individual. This may be information concerning social or private life or state of health. Any data that can directly or indirectly identify a person is considered personal.

The person making the declaration must specify:

• the exact purpose of the file;
• the organization that is keeping the data;
• the organization(s) that produced the data;
• the organization that controls access rights;
• the operating principles of the database;

- measures used to protect the information;
- the type of information managed and the various users; and
- any connection or intended connection with other databases [IFL 1978, art. 14–24].

No computer file (medical or otherwise) may contain information on race, religion, political or philosophical beliefs, or union membership without the expressed authorization of the CNIL and the agreement of the *Conseil d'Etat* [IFL 1978, art. 31].

In the medical field, however, the limitations concerning information on religion or race are often considered as a hindrance to medical activity (e.g., opposition on religious grounds to blood transfusions) or epidemiology research (e.g., the influence of ethnic origins on morbidity), and exceptions have usually been granted. The CNIL may refuse the creation of a computer file or order the partial or total destruction of such files. The CNIL must be notified of any modifications in the purpose, type of information stored, or procedures used. Failure to make any of these declarations, as well as false or incomplete declarations, are punishable by law and may lead to stiff fines and/or prison sentences [IFL 1978, art. 41-44].

Ownership of Medical Records and Access to Personal Information

In a hospital, the medical record belongs neither to patients nor to their physician(s) but to the hospital represented by its director [CSP 1995, art. R.710-2]. The hospital director is responsible for making declarations to the CNIL. Although the director is responsible for the archives (computerized or not), he or she may not access the contents of medical records. This is particularly true for medical information necessary for the program to medicalize information systems [CSP 1995, art. R710-5]. Any correlations made with economic information can only be made on anonymous files.

When a patient is transferred from medical center *A* to center *B*, the electronic transfer of the patient's records may not be handled automatically but only with the consent of the patient and his or her physician(s) at *A*. Center *A* cannot obtain information on the progress of its patients transferred to *B* without the explicit consent of center *B* and the patient.

Medical secrecy does not apply to the patient, who has the right to know any data concerning him. Access to medical records may only be obtained through the physician responsible for the record [IFL 1978, art. 40]. The physician also has the right to keep from the patient any information that might be harmful to him (e.g., a serious diagnosis or a severe prognosis) [CDM 1995, art. 35]. "...in the patient's best interest and for legitimate reasons determined by the physician's conscience, a serious diagnosis or prognosis may be kept from the patient, except in cases where the patient's disease may put others at risk of contamination. A fatal prognosis should only be revealed with circumspection, but the next-of-kin should be notified, unless the patient has previously forbidden this revelation or has designated a third party to be notified instead." This rule, based on the concept of the patient's best interests, is used fairly often in Latin countries, but rarely in Anglo-

Saxon countries, where patients are more readily informed of serious diseases.

For the best interests of the population, secrets concerning diagnoses (infectious diseases that must be reported, accidents at work, professional diseases, etc.) may be revealed to government agencies or to a Social Security agency (e.g., to obtain 100% coverage of certain medical expenses). These exceptions do not apply to life insurance companies, whose interests are not always those of the patient.

These strict regulations have considerably hindered the creation of medical databases for epidemiological research or for improving the knowledge of public health (e.g., public diseases registers). Those responsible for the data were not always involved in treating patients and had knowledge that was covered by medical privacy. The law of July 1, 1994 modified the law of January 6, 1978 to facilitate this kind of research.

Measures Concerning Hardware, Software, and Organization

Those responsible for the files must take the necessary precautions to ensure that the files are protected and data secure. These measures may involve hardware, software, or organization.

Physical Protection of the Files

Figure 15.2 summarizes the basic precautions necessary for physically protecting files.

• Protect computing centers

• Install hardware in protected areas

• Make regular backups of files

• Keep backups in an off-site location

Figure 15.2 : Examples of physical means for protecting data

User Identification

All computer system users must be uniquely identified. This can be done using the keyboard or other methods such as identification cards (e.g., smart cards).

The identification process must also include an authentication process where the user proves he or she is indeed the person identified. This is usually done with passwords. The user is the only person who knows his password, or who can change it. Several unsuccessful attempts to enter the password should automatically block use of the account.

Defining Access and Usage Rights

Access and usage rights are defined by user profiles. These profiles include the user's profession, the types of data the person may access, and the functions or computer programs he or she may use (Figure 15.3).

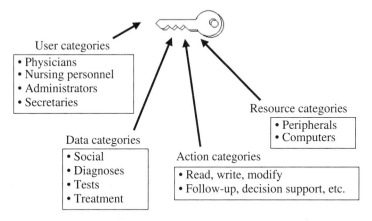

Figure 15.3 : User profiles

Administrative personnels are not authorized to access medical data. Some medical data or permission to modify therapeutic data are only available to certain physicians. This hierarchy of user categories, data, and actions can be associated with resource categories (i.e., terminals, printers, computers, etc.). A user can only access certain types of peripherals at certain times.

Data Encryption

Data encryption encodes information to be stored in such a way that only users with proper authorization may view the encrypted data (Figure 15.4). Even the person responsible for managing the database cannot read the encrypted data. Encryption can be done using software or hardware (e.g., to transmit sensitive data over a network).

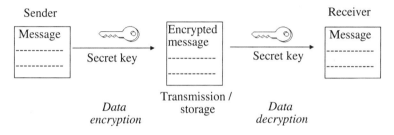

Figure 15.4 : Data encryption principles

Surveillance Programs

The various operations carried out on files containing personal information may be recorded in a transaction log. Besides the dissuasive nature of this type of surveillance, system administrators may supervise access and even trace the source of any illicit break-ins to a computer system. This is particularly important for networks that are accessible from hundreds of peripherals, the telephone network, or public networks such as the Internet [Rind 1997].

Organizational Measures

Besides training and informing personnel on security and secrecy problems, these measures include developing access procedures and appointing individuals responsible for defining the establishment's security regulations.

Discussion and Conclusion

Legislators and health professionals have made considerable efforts to control the risks of protecting individual privacy. Nevertheless, the responsibilities of software developers in the health field must be analyzed and regulated. Although all countries have established procedures for evaluating a therapy or a medical device and determining its advantages, its efficiency, and its dangers, this is not the case for software. Furthermore, the responsibility of the physician or the nurse using a computer system is not always clearly defined. For example, if a technical problem on the hospital's computer network (or in a program) causes a nurse to provide incorrect information to a physician, who is responsible? What is the extent of the hardware manufacturer's responsibility, or that of the software developer? Would the health professional be responsible for errors caused by the use of a computer system? These questions arise for medical record management systems and for computer systems in general that include decision-support programs.

Exercises

- *List some techniques that ensure data integrity in case of hardware failure or software errors.*
- *Discuss the physical and software-based techniques that help ensure data confidentiality.*
- *Cite the major legislation concerning the protection of individuals.*
- *Describe the legal procedure necessary for creating a computer file containing personal information.*
- *Discuss the security issues related to computer networks and the information superhighway.*

Appendix A

Review of Probabilities

Introduction

Probability theory creates models for uncertain processes. It provides useful rules for medical decision support tools.

Uncertain propositions are assigned numeric values indicating their likelihood. These parameters are combined and manipulated according to probability theory and obey the three following axioms:

$$0 \leq P(A) \leq 1 \tag{A.1}$$

$$P(\text{certain}) = 1 \tag{A.2}$$

$$P(A \lor B) = P(A) + P(B) - P(A \land B) \tag{A.3}$$

where $P(A \land B)$ indicates the probability of the joint occurrence of A and B. $P(A \land B)$ equals 0 if A and B are mutually exclusive.

Conditional Probabilities

The basic expressions of the Bayesian formalism are statements on conditional probability. $P(A|B)$ denotes the probability of event A contingent upon the presence of event B. It is equal to:

$$P(A|B) = \frac{P(A \land B)}{P(B)} \tag{A.4}$$

$P(A|B) = P(A)$ if A and B are independent, that is, if the occurrence of A has no influence on the occurrence of B and vice versa.

From equation (A.4) and the equation $P(A \land B) = P(B \land A)$, we can deduce equation (A.5):

$$P(A|B) \cdot P(B) = P(B|A) \cdot P(A) \tag{A.5}$$

Bayes' Formula

Bayes' formula expresses the probability of having a disease (written D) when a sign (written S) is present. The conditional probability of D if S can be deduced from equation (A.5):

$$P(D|S) = \frac{P(S|D) \cdot P(D)}{P(S)} \qquad (A.6)$$

where $P(D)$ represents the *a priori* probability of D.

If we write $\overline{D}$ to indicate the absence of the disease, $P(S|D)$ designates the probability of finding the sign S when the disease is absent. We can express $P(S)$ as a function of the conditional probabilities $P(S|D)$ and $P(S|D)$, that is:

$$P(S) = P(S|D) \cdot P(D) + P(S|D) \cdot P(D) \qquad (A.7)$$

from which we can deduce Bayes' formula:

$$P(D|S) = \frac{P(S|D) \cdot P(D)}{P(S|D) \cdot P(D) + P(S|\overline{D}) \cdot P(\overline{D})} \qquad (A.8)$$

which is generally written:

$$P(D_i|S) = \frac{P(S|D_i) \times P(D_i)}{\sum_i (P(S|D_i) \times P(D_i))} \qquad (A.9)$$

Relative Risk and Odds Ratio

The *odds* of the occurrence of an event E is the ratio of the probability of observing E compared to the probability of not observing it.

$$\text{Odds}_E = \frac{P(E)}{1 - P(E)} \qquad (A.10)$$

The probability of the occurrence of an event E during a given time period t is called the *incidence* of E.

The incidence of an event may be associated with the existence of an endogenous factor F (such as the presence of a genetic marker) or an exogenous factor (such as exposure to a physical condition, or the administration of a drug). Such a factor is called a *risk factor*.

For an event E and a factor F, the comparison of the incidence of E among exposed subjects, or $P(E|F)$, and nonexposed subjects, or $P(E|F)$, may be expressed in several ways:

- The *attributable risk* (AR) of factor F is defined as the difference (or ΔR) between the incidence among exposed subjects and non-exposed subjects:

$$\Delta R \;=\; AR \;=\; P(E|F) - P(E|\bar{F}) \tag{A.11}$$

- The *relative risk* (RR) is defined as the ratio of these two probabilities:

$$RR \;=\; \frac{P(E|F)}{P(E|\bar{F})} \tag{A.12}$$

- The *odds ratio (OR)* associated with factor F, defined as OR_F, is the ratio between the odds of exposed versus nonexposed subjects:

$$OR_F \;=\; \frac{\dfrac{P(E|F)}{1 - P(E|F)}}{\dfrac{P(E|\bar{F})}{1 - P(E|\bar{F})}} \tag{A.13}$$

From equations (A.12) and (A.13) we can deduce

$$RR \;=\; \frac{OR_F}{1 + P(E|\bar{F}) \cdot OR_F} \tag{A.14}$$

The probability of the occurrence of event E in the absence of factor F $P(E|\bar{F})$ is called the *baseline risk*.

If the factor F is a therapeutic procedure, given the baseline risk, the number of patients needed to treat (NNT) to avoid the occurrence of event E equals

$$NNT \;=\; \frac{1}{P(E|\bar{F}) - P(E|F)} \tag{A.15}$$

The NNT can be written as a function of the baseline risk and the RR:

$$NNT \;=\; \frac{1}{P(E|\bar{F}) \cdot (1 - RR)} \tag{A.16}$$

For example, if the probability of death in 5 years is 10% without treatment, and the probability is 8% for patients who received treatment, the absolute reduction in risk is 2%, the relative reduction of risk is 20%, and the number of subjects that must be treated to avoid one death is 50.

Appendix B

Review of Logic

Introduction

In logic, mathematicians have developed formal languages including, among others, propositional logic and predicate logic. Starting from a set of expressions in a symbolic language, and using inference rules, logic can derive new expressions in the language. Two aspects of logic, the syntax and the semantics should be distinguished:

- The syntax defines expressions (or formulas) belonging to the formal language, based on a set of symbols and rules for writing or rewriting.
- Semantics provides a framework for interpreting these formulas, in order to evaluate the conditions in which they are true or false (true and false are two values of truth in classical logic).

Propositional Logic

A *proposition* is a statement, judgment, or expression of a thought. In propositional logic, a proposition can be interpreted as one of the two boolean values *true* T or *false* F. Propositions may be symbolized by letters. We speak of propositions $a, b, \ldots p, q \ldots$.

> Example:
> Proposition a: Diabetes is a chronic disease.
> Proposition b: Diabetes is a frequent disease.

In these two examples, a and b represent *elementary propositions* or atomic formulas. A *compound proposition* or *complex proposition* or *formula* is built from a number n of atomic propositions linked by connectors. Formulas are syntactically correct expressions of the language or propositions. For example, the sentence "Diabetes is a chronic and frequent disease" could be represented by the formula $a \wedge b$.

The four principal connectors are:

- AND (conjunction), written $\wedge$
- OR (disjunction), written $\vee$
- IF...THEN... (implication), written $\supset$ or $\rightarrow$

• IF AND ONLY IF (equivalence), written ≡ or ↔

These connectors are defined by the truth table in Figure B.1. We can note that the implication relationship $p \supset q$ is only false in one situation: where p is true and q is false.

p	q	$p \vee q$	$p \wedge q$	$p \supset q$	$p \equiv q$
F	F	F	F	T	T
F	T	T	F	T	F
T	F	T	F	F	F
T	T	T	T	T	T

Figure B.1 : Truth table for the connectors OR ($\vee$), AND($\wedge$),
IF...THEN... ($\supset$), and ...IF AND ONLY IF... ($\equiv$)

The negation of a proposition p is written $\neg p$. The truth value of $\neg p$ is F when p is interpreted as T and T when p is interpreted as F.

Identity	$p \equiv p$
	$p \supset p$
Non contradiction	$\neg(p \wedge \neg p)$
Commutation	$(p \wedge q) \equiv (q \wedge p)$
	$(p \vee q) \equiv (q \vee p)$
Distribution	$p \wedge (q \vee r) \equiv (p \wedge q) \vee (p \wedge r)$
	$p \vee (q \wedge r) \equiv (p \vee q) \wedge (p \vee r)$
Association	$p \wedge (q \wedge r) \equiv (p \wedge q) \wedge r$
	$p \vee (q \vee r) \equiv (p \vee q) \vee r$
Duality or De Morgan's Theorems	$\neg(p \wedge q) \equiv (\neg p \vee \neg q)$
	$\neg(p \vee q) \equiv (\neg p \wedge \neg q)$
Double negation	$\neg(\neg p) \equiv p$
Implication	$(p \supset q) \equiv (\neg p \vee q)$
Equivalence	$(p \equiv q) \equiv ((p \wedge q) \vee (\neg p \wedge \neg q))$

Figure B.2 : A few properties of connectors (adapted from [Copi 1994])

Connectors have several properties, and several of the most traditional are presented in Figure B.2. They let us rewrite formulas in equivalent forms.

If f is a formula and a, b and c are atoms whose occurrences form f, an interpretation of f is a state where a, b, and c are assigned truth values. If there are n atoms in a formula, there are 2^n possible interpretations for that formula. A formula that is false in all its interpretations is an inconsistent formula, called a *contradiction*. A formula that is true in all of its interpretations is a valid formula, also called a *tautology*.

If $f_1, f_2, ..., f_n, c$ are formulas, c is a *logical consequence* of f_i if and only if, for all interpretations in which $f_1, f_2, ..., f_n$ are true, c is also true. In this case:

• the formula $(f_1 \wedge f_2 \wedge ... \wedge f_n) \supset c$ is a tautology, and

- the formula $(f_1 \wedge f_2 \wedge \ldots \wedge f_n) \wedge \neg c$ is inconsistent.

To be able to deduce the truth value of new formulas from a set of propositions, we need inference rules. Figure B.3 presents different inference rules used in decision support systems. In this figure, the symbol $\therefore$ should be read as "therefore we can formally deduce that".

Modus ponens	$((p \supset q) \wedge p) \therefore q$
Modus tollens	$((p \supset q) \wedge \neg q) \therefore \neg p$
Transitive implication (or hypothetical syllogism)	$((p \supset q) \wedge (q \supset r)) \therefore (p \supset r)$
Disjunctive syllogism	$((p \vee q) \wedge \neg p) \therefore q$
Reduction to the absurd	$((p \supset q) \wedge (p \supset \neg q)) \therefore \neg p$
Simplification	$(p \wedge q) \therefore p$
Addition	$p \therefore (p \vee q)$

Figure B.3 : A few rules of inference

The inference rule *modus ponens* (from the Latin *pono*, to affirm) is expressed as follows:

If the proposition p is true and if $p \supset q$ we can formally deduce that the proposition q is true.

The inference rule *modus tollens* (from the Latin *tollo*, to deny) is expressed as follows:

If the proposition q is false and if $p \supset q$, we can formally deduce that the proposition p is false.

Predicate Logic

Also known as *first-order logic*, this is an extension of propositional logic. It introduces the concept of variables, quantifiers, and functions. If the symbols (other than connectors) that make up the alphabet of propositional logic are reduced to propositions themselves, the first-order language is more complex. It includes constants, variables, connectors, quantifiers, relational symbols (predicates), and functional symbols.

A *variable* is a subset of the authorized symbols in a domain that takes its values from the set of all constants. Variables are normally represented in lowercase letters $x,$ y or z.

Quantifiers specify how a formula is to be evaluated by indicating the particular conditions of the variables. We may define two quantifiers:

- the *universal quantifier* (for any), written $\forall$, and
- the *existential quantifier* (there is), written $\exists$.

A *function* is an application of the set of all constants to itself (e.g., $f(x)$).

A *predicate* is an application of the set of all constants in the set {T, F} that is a propositional function of a domain towards a truth value. If the domain includes n variables, where $n = 0, 1, 2, \ldots$, the function is called a predicate with n positions (e.g., $P(x, y)$). A proposition is a predicate where $n = 0$. Predicates can assign properties (attributes) to objects. In the phrase "Herman is ill", Herman is the subject and ill is the predicate. The predicate $D(x)$, which may symbolically represent the function $disease(x)$, is neither true nor false. The truth value depends on each instance of x. The formula $\forall x P(x)$ indicates that $P(x)$ is true for all instances of x. The formula $\exists x P(x)$ indicates there is at least one instance of x for which $P(x)$ is true.

Examples:

- Herman, 1, 2, and Ohio are constants.
- x, glycemia, and address are variables.
- Ideal-weight(x) is a function.
- Father(Herman) is a predicate to an instance of a variable that has the value of "Herman".
- Brother(x, Herman) is a predicate with two variables, the first of which is free and the second of which has an instance of "Herman".
- $\forall x P(x)$ is a formula of the first order universally quantified (e.g., example, $\forall x \text{Mortal}(x)$: everything is mortal).

The concepts of the interpretation of formulas and of the logical consequences presented in propositional logic extend to first-order logic. The PROLOG programming language, widely used in artificial intelligence, is based on first-order logic.

Appendix C

Some Useful References

Medical Informatics Associations

In France

The Association for applications of Informatics in Medicine (AIM) was created in 1968. This association is made up of different work groups debating various themes dealing with computers in medicine. It organizes two annual conferences. Conferences proceedings are published in the collection "Informatique et Santé" by Springer-Verlag (France). The address of the current president is:

> Professeur Régis Beuscart
> Laboratoire d'Informatique Médicale
> Faculté de Médecine
> 1 Place de Verdun 59045 Lille, France
>
> E-mail: rbeuscart@chru-lille.fr
> URL: http://www.hbroussais.fr/Broussais/InforMed/AIM.html

In Europe

The associations for medical computing in European countries are grouped together in a federation: the European Federation for Medical Informatics. The EFMI organizes an annual conference (except for the year of the MED-INFO, organized by the IMIA). The address of the current president is:

> Prof. Jean Raoul Scherrer
> Département d'Informatique Médicale
> Hôpital cantonal de Genève
> 1211 Geneva 14, Switzerland
>
> E-mail: scherrer@cih.hcuge.ch
> URL: http://www.eur.nl/FGG/MI/imia/home.html

In the United States

The American Medical Informatics Association (AMIA) organizes the annual SCAMC conference. The address of the AMIA office is:

AMIA Office:
4915 St. Elmo Avenue, Suite 401
Bethesda, MD 20814 USA

E-mail: mail@amia2.amia.org
URL: http://amia2.amia.org/

The International Medical Informatics Association

The International Medical Informatics Association (IMIA) is the worldwide
organization that groups representatives from the various country organizations. It organizes the MEDINFO conference every three years. The address
of the current president is:

Prof. Jan H. van Bemmel
Dept of Medical Informatics
Faculty of Medicine and Health Services
Erasmus University PO Box 1738 Rotterdam, The Netherlands

E-mail: vanbemmel@mi.fgg.eur.nl
URL: http://www.imia.org/

Principal International Conferences

MEDINFO

The IMIA organizes the worldwide medical informatics conference (MED-
INFO) every three years. The conference proceedings have been published
by Elsevier North Holland (Amsterdam) and IOS Press (Amsterdam).

SCAMC- AMIA fall symposium

The AMIA organizes a fall symposium formerly Symposium on Computer
Applications in Medical Care (SCAMC). The conference notes were published by the IEEE in Washington until 1993. They are now published as a
supplement to the *Journal of the American Medical Informatics Association*
(JAMIA).

EFMI Conference

The EFMI organizes the annual Medical Informatics Europe (MIE), except
in the years of the MEDINFO. The conference proceedings are published by
IOS Press (Amsterdam).

Principal Specialized Publications

• *Artificial Intelligence in Medicine* (Amsterdam: Elsevier)

- *Computers in Biology and Medicine* (Oxford: Pergamon Press)
- C*omputers in Biomedical Research* (San Diego: Academic Press)
- *Computer Methods and Programs in Biomedicine* (Amsterdam: Elsevier)
- *IEEE Engineering in Medicine and Biology Magazine* (New York: IEEE)
- *IEEE Transactions on Biomedical Engineering* (New York: IEEE)
- *International Journal of Medical Informatics* (Limerick: Elsevier)
- *Journal of Medical System*s (New York: Plenum Press)
- *Journal of the American Medical Informatics Association* (Philadelphia: Hanley & Belfus)
- *MD Computing* (New York: Springer-Verlag)
- *Medical Informatics & The Internet in Medicine* (London: Taylor & Francis)
- *Methods of Information in Medicine* (Stuttgart: Schattauer)
- *Yearbook of Medical Informatics* (Stuttgart: Schattauer) Annual selection of key articles in medical informatics.

Internet Addresses

General Catalogs and Electronic Libraries

General catalogs of Internet sites, including biology and health.

> http://galaxy.einet.net/galaxy.html
> http://golgi.harvard.edu/
> http://www.hon.ch/home.html
> http://www.med-library.com/medlibrary/
> http://www.ohsu.edu/cliniweb/wwwvl/
> http://www-sci.lib.uci.edu/HSG/HSGuide.html

Informatics in Health Care and Telemedicine, Standards

> http://www.chu-rouen.fr/ssm/watch.html
> http://www.imbi.uni-freiburg.de/medinf/mi_list.htm
> http://www.mcis.duke.edu/standards/guide.htm
> http://www.cpmc.columbia.edu/edu/textbook/

Medical Informatics Textbooks

Introduction to Clinical Informatics

> http://www.hbroussais.fr/clininform/

Handbook of Medical Informatics

> http://www.mieur.nl/mihandbook/

Data and Knowledge Banks

NLM

The National Library of Medicine maintains 40 bibliographical databases and databanks including MEDLINE (see Chapter 6).

> http://www.nlm.nih.gov/
> http://www.ncbi.nlm.nih.gov/PubMed/

Bioinformatics

> http://www.corse.inra.fr/sra/servbiol.htm
> http://www.embl-heidelberg.de/
> http://www.ebi.ac.uk/
> http://www.expasy.ch/
> http://www.ncbi.nlm.nih.gov/Web/Genbank/index.html
> http://gdbwww.gdb.org/

Medical guidelines, Evidence-Based Medicine

COCHRANE

Databank covering several thousands therapeutic trials.

> http://hiru.mcmaster.ca/cochrane/

CPG InfoBase

Clinical Practice Guidelines of the Canadian Medical Association

> http://www.cma.ca/cpgs/index.asp

HSTAT

Electronic resource that provides access to the full-text of documents useful in health care decision making. It includes clinical practice guidelines, quick-reference guides, and evidence reports.

> http://text.nlm.nih.gov/
> http://www.ahcpr.gov/

Bibliography

[Allaert 1996] Allaert FA and Dusserre L. Dossier médical informatisé: déontologie et législation. *Revue du Praticien* 1996; 46: 333–7.

[AMA 1999] *CPT 1999*. American Medical Association, 515 north State Street, Chicago (IL 60610) 1998.

[Aronow 1988] Aronow DB. Severity of Illness Measurement: Applications in quality assurance and utilization review. *Medical Care Review* 1988; 45(2): 339–66.

[Arsac 1983] Arsac J. *Les bases de la programmation*. Paris: Dunod, 1983.

[Ball 1980] Ball MJ and Jacobs SE. Information systems: the status of level 1. *Hospitals* 1980; 54(12): 179-86.

[Barnett 1984] Barnett GO. The application of computer based medical record systems in ambulatory practice. *New Engl J Med*. 1984; 310: 1643–50.

[Baud 1992] Baud RH, Rassinoux AM, and Scherrer JR. Natural language processing and semantical representation of medical texts. *Methods Inf Med* 1992; 31(2): 117–25.

[Bentsen 1976] Bentsen BG. The accuracy of recording patient problems in family practice. *Journal of Medical Education* 1976; 51: 311.

[Bergeron 1989] Bergeron B and Greenes RA. Skill-building simulations in cardiology: HeartLab and EKGLab. *Comp Meth Prog Biomed* 1989; 30: 111–25.

[Béraud 1995] Béraud Cl. La régulation du système de soins. *Courrier de l'Evaluation en Santé* 1995; 4: 2–24.

[Berwick 1989] Berwick DM. Continuous improvement as an ideal in health care. *New Engl J Med* 1989; 320: 53–6.

[Beuscart 1996] Beuscart R, Ghosn N, and Haye MP. Cartes à microprocesseur et dossier médical portable. *Revue du Praticien* 1996; 46: 314–8.

[Billault 1995] Billault B, Degoulet P, Devriès C, Plouin PF, Chatellier G, and Ménard J. Use of a standardized personal medical record by patients with hypertension: a randomized controlled prospective trial. *MD Computing* 1995; 12 (1): 31–35.

[Bouhaddou 1995] Bouhaddou O and Warner H. An interactive patient information and education system (Medical HouseCall) based on a physician expert system (Iliad). *Medinfo* (Canada), 1995; 8 Pt 2: 1181–5.

[Brewster 1985] Brewster AC, Karlin BG, Hyde LA, Jacobs CM, Bradbury RC, Chae YM. MEDISGRPS: a clinically based approach to classifying hospital patients at admission. *Inquiry* 1985; 22(4): 377–87.

[Brown 1998] Brown PJB, O'Neil M, Price C. Semantic definition of disorders in version 3 of the Read codes. *Meth Inform Med* 1998; 37: 415–9.

[Brunswick 1952] Brunswick E. The Conceptual framework of psychology. In *International Encyclopedia of Unified Science* (Vol. 1, n°10). Chicago: University of Chicago Press, 1952.

[Campbell 1998] Campbell KE, Oliver DE, Spackman KA, Shortliffe EH. Representing thoughts, words, and things in the UMLS. *J Am Med Inform Assoc* 1998; 5(5): 421–31.

[Calore 1987] Calore K and Iezzoni L. Disease staging and PMCs: can they improve DRGs ? *Medical Care* 1987; 25(8).

[Cattel 1994] Cattel RGG. *Object Data Management*. (Revised edition). Reading, Massachusetts: Addison Wesley, 1994.

[CDAM 1985] CDAM. *Catalogue des Actes Médicaux*, Bulletin Officiel n° 85/9bis. Paris: Ministère des Affaires Sociales et de la Solidarité, 1985.

[CDM 1995] *Code de déontologie médicale* (Décret No 95-1000 du 6 Septembre 1995).

[Chatellier 1996] Chatellier G, Zapletal E, Lemaitre D, Ménard J, and Degoulet P. The number needed to treat : a clinically useful nomogram in its proper context. *Br Med J* 1996; 312: 426–9.

[CE 1981] Conseil de l'Europe. *Recommandation No (81)1 du comité des ministres aux Etats membres relative à la réglementation applicable aux banques de données médicales automatisées.* 23 Janvier 1981.

[Cherrak 1997] Cherrak I, Paul JF, jaulent MC, Chatellier G, plouin PF, Gaux JC, Degoulet P. Automatic stenosis detection and quantification in renal arteriography. *Proc AMIA Annu Fall Symp.* 1997; pp. 66–70.

[Chute 1992] Chute CG. Clinical data retrieval and analysis. I've seen a case like that before. *Ann N Y Acad Sci* 1992; 670: 133–40.

[CIOM 1987] Conférence Internationale des Ordres et des Organismes d'Attributions Similaires. *Principes d'éthique médicale européenne.* Paris, 1987.

[Cimino 1994] Cimino JJ, Clayton PD, Hripcsak G, and Johnson SB. Knowledge-based approaches to the maintenance of a large controlled medical terminology. *JAMIA* 1994; 1(1): 35–50.

[Cimino 1995] Cimino JJ, Socratous SA, and Clayton PD. Internet as clinical information system: using the World Wide Web. *JAMIA* 1995; 2(5): 273–284.

[Cinquin 1996] Cinquin P. Imagerie médicale et interventions assistées par ordinateur. *Revue du Praticien*, 1996: 46: 319–23.

[Clancey 1986] Clancey WJ. From GUIDON to NEOMYCIN to HERACLES in twenty short lessons. *AI Magazine* 1986; 7(3): 40–50.

[Clancey 1987] Clancey WJ. *Knowledge-based tutoring: the GUIDON program*. Cambridge, MA: MIT Press 1987.

[Clayton 1989] Clayton PD, Pryor AT, Wigertz OB, and Hripcsak G. Issues and structures for sharing medical knowledge among decision-making systems: the 1989 Arden Homestead retreat. *Proc Annu Symp Comput Appl Med Care* 1989; pp. 116–21.

[Clyman 1990] Clyman SG and Orr NA. Status report on the NBME's computer-based testing. *Acad Med* 1990, 65(4): 235–41.

[Codd 1990] Codd EF. *The Relational Model for Database Management*. Version 2. Reading, Massachusetts: Addison Wesley, 1990.

[Copi 1994] Copi IM and Cohen C. *Introduction to Logic*. New York: Macmillan Publishing Company, 1994.

[Côté 1993] Côté RA, Rothwell DJ, Beckett RS, Palotay JL, and Brochu L (eds). *SNOMED International* (4 volumes). Northfield: College of American Pathologists (325 Waukegan Road, Northfield, IL 60093-2650, Phone: 708/446-8800), 1993.

[CP 1995] *Code pénal*. Paris: Dalloz (11, rue Soufflot, Paris 75005), 1995–1996.

[CSP 1995] *Code de la santé publique. Code de la famille et de l'aide sociale*. Paris: Dalloz (11, rue Soufflot, Paris 75005), 1995.

[Cundick 1989] Cundick R, Turner C, Lincoln M, Buchanan J, Anderson C, Warner H, and Bouhaddou O. Iliad as a patient case simulator to teach medical problem solving. *Proc Annu Symp Comput Appl Med Care* (13th SCAMC) 1989, pp. 902–6.

[Date 1995] Date CJ. *An Introduction to Database Systems*. Sixth edition. Reading, Mass.: Addison Wesley, 1995.

[Davis 1991] Davis S and Davidson B. *2020 vision*. New York: Simon & Schuster, 1991.

[de Dombal 1979] de Dombal FT. Computers and the surgeon: a matter of Decision. *Surg Ann* 1979; 11: 33–57.

[De Moor 1993] De Moor G, McDonald CJ, and Noothoven van Goor J (eds). *Progress in Standardization in Health Care Informatics*. Amsterdam: IOS Press, 1993.

[De Moor 1995] De Moor G. European standards development in healthcare informatics: actual and future challenges. *Int J Biomed Comput* 1995; 39: 81–5.

[Degoulet 1986] Degoulet P, Devriès C, Rioux P, Chantalou JP, Klinger E, Sauquet D, Zweigenbaum P, and Aimé F. LIED : a temporal data base management system. In: R. Salamon, B. Blum, M. Jorgensen (eds). *Proceedings MEDINFO 86*. Amsterdam : North-Holland. 1986; pp. 532–6.

[Degoulet 1989] Degoulet P and Jean FC. Pragmatic database modeling. In: B. Barber, D. Cao, D. Qin, G. Wagner (eds). *Proceedings MEDINFO 89*. Amsterdam : North-Holland. 1989; pp.1127–31.

[Degoulet 1990] Degoulet P, Chatellier G, Devriès C, Lavril M, and Ménard J. Computer assisted techniques for evaluation and treatment of hypertensive patients. *Am J Hypertension* 1990; 3:156–63.

[Degoulet 1995] Degoulet P, Fieschi M, and Chatellier G. Decision support systems from the standpoint of knowledge representation. *Meth Inform Med* 1995; 34: 202–8.

[Dick 1991] Dick RS and Steen EB (eds). *The Computerized-Based Patient Record. An Essential Technology for Health Care – Institute of Medicine.* Washington, DC: National Academy Press, 1991.

[Doré 1995] Doré L, Lavril M, Jean FC, and Degoulet P. An object-oriented computer-based patient record reference model. *Proc Annu Symp Comput Appl Med Care* 1995; pp. 377–81.

[Dolin 1998] Dolin RH, Rishel W, Biron PV, Spinosa J, Mattison JE. SGML and XML as interchange formats for HL7 messages. *Proc AMIA Annu Fall Symp.* 1997; pp. 590–4.

[Dorenfest 1995] Dorenfest S. *Health Care Information Systems. State of the Art 1995.* Chicago: Dorenfest S & Associates, 1995.

[Ducrot 1989] Ducrot H, Leclerc F, Medernach C, Plotkine M, Trinchet JC, and Vincens O. La banque d'informations automatisées sur les médicaments (BIAM). *Informatique et Santé* (Paris: Springer-Verlag) 1989; 2: 201–7.

[EP 1995] Directive du Parlement Européen et du Conseil du 24 octobre 1995 – Directive 95/46/CE relative à la protection des personnes physiques à l'égard du traitement des données à caractère personnel et à la libre circulation de ces données.

[Engelmann 1995] Engelmann U, Meinzer HP, Schroter A, Gunnel U, Demiris AM, Makabe M, Evers H, Jean FC, and Degoulet P. The image related services of the HELIOS software engineering environment. *Comput Methods Programs Biomed* 1995, 46(1): 1–12.

[Enning 1994] Enning CJ, van Gennip EM, van den Broeck R, Rechid R, Wein B, and Bakker AR. PACER: a software tool for PACS decision makers. *Med Inf* 1994, 19(2): 179–87.

[Evans 1985] Evans RS, Gardner RM, and Bush AR. Development of a Computerized Infectious Disease Monitor (CIDM). *Comput Biomed Res* 1985; 18: 103–13.

[Fetter 1980] Fetter RB, Shin Y, Freeman JL, Averill RF, and Thompson JD. Case mix definition by diagnosis-related groups. *Med Care* 1980: 18 (2 Suppl) piii: 1–53.

[Fieschi 1986] Fieschi M. *Intelligence artificielle en médecine: des systèmes experts*. Paris: Masson, 1986.

[Fieschi 1990] Fieschi M. Towards validation of expert systems as medical decision aids. *Int J Biomed Comput* 1990; 26: 93–108.

[Freeman 1995] Freeman JL, Fetter RB, Park H, Schneider KC, Lichtenstein JL, Hughes JS, Bauman WA, Duncan CC, Freeman DH, and Palmer GR. Diagnosis-related group refinement with diagnosis- and procedure-specific comorbidities and complications. *Med Care* 1995; 33(8): 806–27.

[Frutiger 1991] Frutiger P and Fessler JM. *La gestion hospitalière médicalisée*. Paris: ESF, 1991.

[Gardner 1990a] Gardner RM. Patient monitoring systems. In: *Medical Informatics. Computer Applications in health care*. In: Shortliffe EH, Perreault LE, Wiederhold G, Fagan LM (eds). Reading, Massachusetts: Addison-Wesley 1990: pp. 366–99.

[Gardner 1990b] Gardner RM, Hulse RK, and Larsen KG. Assessing the Effectiveness of a Computerized Pharmacy System. *Proc Annu Symp Comput Appl Med Care* (14th SCAMC) 1990; pp. 668–72.

[Gonella 1984] Gonella JS, Hornbrook MC, Louis DZ. Staging of disease: *JAMA* 1984; 251: 637–44.

[Gonzalez 1992] Gonzalez RC and Woods RE. *Digital Image Processing*. Reading, Mass.: Addison-Wesley, 1992.

[Goupy 1976] Goupy F, Hirel JC, Bloch P, and Berger C. CHRONOS: a database management package for physicians and researchers. *Comp Prog Biomed* 1976; 6: 149–65.

[Grémy 1987] Grémy F. *Informatique Médicale*. Paris: Flammarion. 1987; pp. 49–70.

[Griesser 1977] Griesser GG. Scope and purpose. In: *Realization of data protection in health information systems*. Griesser (ed). Amsterdam: North-Holland. 1977; pp. 1–6.

[Hakansson 1989] Hakansson H. *Corporate technological behavior: cooperation and networks*. London: Routledge, 1989.

[Halamka 1997] Halamka JD, Szolovits P, Rind D, Safran CA WWW implementation of national recommendations for protecting electronic health information. *J Am Med Inform Assoc* 1997; 4(6): 458–64.

[Hammond 1990] Hammond JE, Berger RG, Carey TS, Rutledge R, Cleveland TJ, Kichak JP, and Ayscue CF. Making the transition from information systems of the 1970s to medical information systems of the 1990s: the role of the physician's workstation. *J Med Systems* 1991; 15: 257–67.

[Hammond 1986] Hammond WE and Stead WW. The evolution of a computerized Medical Information System (GEMISH and TMR). *Proc Annu Symp Comput Appl Med Care* 1986; pp. 147–56.

[Hammond 1995] Hammond WE. The status of healthcare standards in the United States. *Int J Biomed Comput* 1995;3 9(1): 87–92.

[Harmon 1985] Harmon P and King D. *Expert systems: Artificial Intelligence in Business.* New York: John Wiley, 1985.

[Harless 1986] Harless WG, Zier MA, and Duncan RC. A voice-activated, interactive videodisc case study for use in the medical school classroom. *J Med Educ* 1986, 61(11): 913–5.

[Hickam 1985] Hickam DH, Shortliffe EH, Bischoff MB, Scott AC, and Jacobs CD. The treatment advice of a computer-based cancer chemotherapy protocol advisor. *Ann Intern Med* 1985, 103 (6 (Pt 1)): 928–36.

[Horn 1983] Horn SD, Sharkey PD, Bertram DA. Measuring severity of illness: homogeneous case mix groups. *Med Care 1983; 21(1): 14–30.*

[Horn 1991] Horn SD, Sharkey PD, Buckle JM, Backofen JE, Averill RF, Horn RA. The relationship between severity of illness and hospital length of stay and mortality. *Med Care 1991; 29(4): 305–17.*

[Hripcsak 1994] Hripcsak G, Ludemann P, Pryor TA, Wigertz OB, and Clayton PD. Rationale for the Arden Syntax. *Comput Biomed Res* 1994; 27(4): 291-324.

[Hunter 1993] Hunter L (ed). *Artificial intelligence and molecular biology.* Menlo Park, CA: AAAI Press, 1993.

[ICD 9 CM 1994] *ICD.9.CM – International Classification of Diseases, 9th Revision, Clinical Modification, Fourth Revision.* Los Angeles: Practice Management Information Corporation, 1994.

[Iezzoni 1997]. Iezzoni LI. The risks of risk adjustment. *JAMA* 1997; 278: 1600–7.

[IFL 1978] Loi No 78-17 du 6 janvier 1978 relative à l'informatique, aux fichiers et aux libertés. *Journal Officiel de la République Française.* pp. 227-231. Décret d'application No 78-774 du 17 juillet 1978, pp. 2906–7.

[ISIS4 1995] ISIS4 Collaborative Group. International Study of Infarction Survival 4 (ISIS4): a randomized factorial trial assessing early oral captopril, oral mononitrate and intravenous magnesium sulfate in 58050 patients with suspected acute myocardial infarction. *Lancet* 1995; 345: 669–85.

[JO 1993] Loi réglementant la transmission des données médicales nominatives au responsable du Département de l'Information Médicale dans le cadre du PMSI. *Journal Officiel de la République Française*, Paris, 27 Janvier 1993.

[Knaus 1985] Knaus WA, Draper EA, Wagner DP, and Zimmerman JE. APACHE II: a severity of disease classification system. *Critical Care Medicine* 1985; 13(10): 818–29.

[Knaus 1991] Knaus WA, Wagner DP, Draper EA, Zimmerman JE, Bergner M, Bastos PG, Sirio CA, Murphy DJ, Lotring T, Damiano A, et al. The APACHE III prognostic system. Risk prediction of hospital mortality for critically ill hospitalized adults. *Chest* 1991;100(6): 1619–36

[Kohane 1996] Kohane IS, van Wingerde FJ, Fackler JC, Cimino C, Szolovits P. W3-EMR : Building national electronic medical record systems via the World Wide Web. *J Am Med Inform Assoc* 1996; 3 : 191–207.

[Laquey 1995] Laquey T. *The European Internet Companion*. Reading, Massachusetts: Addison-Wesley, 1995.

[Launois 1986] Launois RJ and Truchet D. Vers une implantation des réseaux de soins coordonnés. Objectifs économiques et problèmes juridiques. *Journal d'Economie Médicale* 1986; 4(3-4): 155–189.

[Laurière 1987] Laurière JL. *Intelligence Artificielle: résolution de problèmes par l'homme et la machine*. Paris: Eyrolles, 1987.

[Lenoir 1981] Lenoir P, Roger MJ, Frangerel C, and Chales G. Réalisation développement et maintenance de la banque de données ADM. *Med Informatics* 1981; 6: 51–6.

[Lemaitre 1989] Lemaitre P and Maquère F. *Savoir apprendre*. Paris: Chotard, 1989.

[Lemaitre 1994] Lemaitre D, Jaulent MC, Günnel U, Demiris AM, Michel PA, Rassinoux AM, Göransson B, Olsson E, and Degoulet P. ARTEMIS-2: an application development experiment with the HELIOS environment. *Comput Methods Programs Biomed*. 1994; 45, Suppl. : S127–38.

[Lepage 1991] Lepage EF, Gardner RM, Laub RM, and Jacobson JT. Assessing the effectiveness of a computerized blood order "consultation" system. *Proc Annu Symp Comput Appl Med Care* 1991; pp. 33-7.

[Ligier 1994] Ligier Y, Ratib O, Logean M, and Girard C. Osiris: a medical image-manipulation system. *MD Computing* 1994; 11(4): 212–8.

[Lindberg 1993] Lindberg DAB, Humphreys BL, and McCray AT. The Unified Medical Language System. *Meth Inform Med* 1993; 32: 281–91.

[Lohr 1990] Lohr KN, ed. *Medicare: A Strategy for Quality Assurance*. Washington, DC: National Academy Press; 1990.

[McCray 1989] McCray AT. The UMLS Semantic Network. *Proc Annu Symp Comput Appl Med Care* (13th SCAMC) 1989; pp. 503–7.

[McCray 1998] McCray AT. The nature of lexical knowledge. *Meth Inform Med* 1998; 37: 353–60.

[McDonald 1976] McDonald CJ. Protocol-based computers reminders, the quality of care and the non-perfectibility of man. *N Engl J Med* 1976; 295: 1351–5.

[McDonald 1988] McDonald CJ and Tierney WM. Computer-stored medical records. *JAMA* 1988; 259: 3433–40.

[Meinzer 1990] Meinzer HP, Engelmann U, Scheppelmann D, and Schäfer R. Volume visualization of 3D tomographies. In: *3D Imaging in Medicine*. Höhne KH et al. (eds). NATO ASI Series, Vol. F60. Berlin: Springer-Verlag, 1990: pp. 253–61.

[Meinzer 1996] Meinzer HP and Engelmann U. Medical images in integrated health care workstations. In: JH van Bemmel, AT McCray (eds). *Yearbook of Medical Informatics* 1996. Stuttgart: Schattauer, 1996; pp. 87–94.

[MeSH 1999] Medical Subject Headings, 1999 Supplement to Index Medicus. (U.S. Government Printing Office. National Technical Information Service, U.S. Department of Commerce, Springfield, VA 22161), 1999.

[Miller 1982] Miller RA, Pople H, and Myers J. INTERNIST-1: An experimental computer-based diagnostic consultant for general internal medicine. *N Engl J Med* 1982; 307: 468–76.

[Miller 1986a] Miller P. *Expert Critiquing Systems: Practice-Based Medical Consultation by Computer.* New York: Springer-Verlag, 1986.

[Miller 1986b] Miller RA, McNeil MA, Challinor SM, Masarie FE, and Myers JD. The Internist-1/Quick Medical Reference project–status report. *West J Med* 1986; 145(6): 816–22.

[Miller 1994] Miller RA. Medical diagnostic decision support systems — past, present, and future: a threaded bibliography and brief commentary. *J Am Med Inform Assoc* 1994; 1(1): 8–27.

[Minsky 1975] Minsky M. A Framework for Representing Knowledge. In: P. Winston (ed). *The psychology of computer vision.* New York: McGraw-Hill, 1975: pp. 211–77.

[MRI 1988] Ministère de l'Industrie, des P & T et du Tourisme. *RACINES, schéma directeur de l'informatique.* Vol 1. Manuel des dirigeants. Vol. 2. Manuel de réalisation. Paris: La Documentation française, 1988.

[Nakao 1983] Nakao MA and Axelrod S. Number are better than words: Verbal specifications of frequency have no place in medicine. *Am J Med* 1983: 74: 1061–5.

[Nanci 1992] Nanci D, Espinasse B, Cohen B, and Heckenroth H. *Ingénierie des systèmes d'information avec Merise.* Paris: Sybex, 1992.

[NHS 1995] *The Read Codes – Version 3.* NHS Center for Coding and Classification (Woodgate, LE11 2TG, UK).

[OMS 1977] OMS. *Classification internationale des Maladies*. Neuvième révision. Genève: Organisation Mondiale de la Santé, 1977.

[Pauker 1976] Pauker SG, Gorry GA, Kassirer JP, Schwartz WB. Towards the simulation of clinical cognition. Taking a present illness by computer. *Am J Med* 1976; 60: 981–96.

[Philbrick 1980] Philbrick JT, Horwitz RI, and Feinstein AR. Methodologic problems of exercise testing for coronary disease: groups, analysis, and bias. *Am J Cardiol* 1980: 46: 807–12.

[Pryor 1987] Pryor TA, Clayton PD, Haug PJ, and Wigertz O. Design of a know ledge driven HIS. *Proc Annu Symp Comput Appl Med Care* (11th SCAMC) 1987: 60–3.

[Pryor 1988] Pryor AT. The HELP medical record system. *MD Computing* 1988; 5(5): 22–33.

[Rassinoux 1995] Rassinoux AM, Wagner J, Lovis C, Baud R, Rector A, and Scherrer JR. Analysis of medical texts based on a sound medical model. *Proc Annu Symp Comput Appl Med Care* (19th SCAMC) 1995; pp. 27–31.

[Rassinoux 1998] Rassinoux AM, Miller RA, Baud RH, Scherrer JR. Modeling concepts in medicine for medical language understanding. *Meth Inform Med* 1998; 37: 361–72.

[Ratib 1994] Ratib O, Ligier Y, and Scherrer JR. Digital image management and communication in medicine. *Comput Med Imaging Graph* 1994, 18(2): 73–84.

[RCGP 1984] RCGP (Royal College of General Practitioners). New Classification of Diseases and Problems. *J R Coll Gen Pract* 1984; 34: 125–7.

[Rector 1994] Rector AL. The GALEN project. *Comp Methods Programs Biomed*. 1994; 45(1-2): 75–8.

[Rind 1995] Rind DM, Davis R, and Safran C. Designing studies of computer-based alerts and reminders. *MD Computing* 1995; 12: 122–6.

[Rind 1997] Rind DM, Kohane IS, Szolovits P, Safran C, Chueh HC, Barnett GO. Maintaining the confidentiality of medical records shared over the Internet and the World Wide Web. *Ann Intern Med* 1997; 127: 138–41.

[Robert 1994] *Le Nouveau Petit Robert*. Paris: Dictionnaires le Robert, 1994.

[Safran 1989] Safran CD, Porter D, Lightfoot J, Rury CD, Underhill LH, Bleich HL, and Slack WV. ClinQuery: a system for on-line searching of data in a teaching hospital. *Ann Int Med* 1989; 111: 751–6.

[Safran 1994] Safran C. Defining clinical workstations. *Int J Biomed Comput*, 1994; 34: 261–265.

[Safran 1995] Safran C and Chute CG. Exploration and exploitation of clinical databases. *Int J Biomed Comput* 1995; 39(1): 151–6.

[Scherrer 1990] Scherrer JR, Baud R, Hochstrasser D, and Ratib O. An integrated hospital information system. *Medical Computing* 1990; 7: 81–9.

[Schwartz 1986] Schwartz S and Griffin T. *Medical Thinking: The Psychology of Medical Judgment and Decision Making.* New-York: Springer Verlag, 1986.

[Sheiner 1972] Sheiner LB, Rosenberg B, and Melmon KL. Modelling of individual pharmacokinetics for computer-aided drug dosage. *Computer Biomed Res* 1972; 5: 441–59.

[Shortliffe 1976] Shortliffe EH. *Computer-Based Medical Consultation: MYCIN.* New York: American Elsevier, 1976.

[Shortliffe 1986] Shortliffe EH. Medical expert systems--knowledge tools for physicians. *West J Med* 1986; 145(6): 830–9.

[Shortliffe 1990] Shortliffe EH, Perreault LE, Wiederhold G, and Fagan LM (eds). *Medical Informatics. Computer applications in health care.* Reading, Massachusetts: Addison-Wesley, 1990.

[Silvermann 1991] Silvermann B. *Modeling and critiquing Human error: A Knowledge Based Human-Computer Collaboration Approach.* Book draft, Student Coop G. Washington University, 1991.

[Stewart 1998] Integration of DICOM images into an electronic medical record using thin viewing clients. *Proc AMIA Annu Fall Symp.* 1998; pp. 902–6.

[Smith 1994] Smith DW (ed). *Biocomputing. Informatics and the Genome Project.* San Diego, CA: Academic Press, 1994.

[Sowa 1984] Sowa JF. *Conceptual Structures. Information processing in mind and machine.* Reading, MA: Addison-Wesley, 1984.

[Spackman 1997] Spackman KA, Campbell KE, Cote RA. SNOMED RT: a reference terminology for health care. *Proc AMIA Annu Fall Symp.* 1997; pp. 640–4.

[Sprague 1992] Sprague D. How will multimedia change system storage. *Byte* 1992; 17(3): 165–6.

[Tapscott 1993] Tapscott D and Caston A. *Paradigm shift. The new promise of information technology.* New York: McGraw-Hill, 1993.

[UMLS 1996] *UMLS Knowledge Source.* 7th Experimental Edition. Bethesda (MD) : NLM/NIH (8600 Rockville Pike, Bethesda 20864, USA), January 1996.

[Valleron 1993] Valleron AJ and Garnerin P. Computerised surveillance of communicable diseases in France. *Commun Dis Rep CDR Rev* 1993; 3(6): R82–7.

[Van Bemmel 1992] van Bemmel JH, Kors JA, and van Herpen G. Combination of diagnostic classifications from ECG and VCG computer interpretations. *J Electrocardiol* 1992, 25 Suppl: 126–30.

[Van Bemmel 1997] van Bemmel JH, Musen MA. *Handbook of Medical Informatics*. Heidelberg: Springer, 1997; pp. 399–411.

[Van de Velde 1992] van de Velde R. *Hospital Information Systems. The next generation*. Berlin: Springer-Verlag, 1992.

[Van Mulligen 1995] van Mulligen E, Cornet R, Timmers T. Problems with integrating legacy systems. *Proc Annu Symp Comput Appl Med Care* 1995; 747–51.

[Warner 1988] Warner HR, Haug P, Bouhaddou O, Lincoln M, Warner H, Sorenson D, Williamson JW, and Fan C. ILIAD as an expert consultant to teach differential diagnosis. *Proc Annu Symp Comput Appl Med Care* (12th SCAMC) 1988; pp. 371–6.

[Waterman 1986] Waterman DA. *A Guide to Expert Systems*. Reading, Massachusetts: Addison-Wesley, 1986.

[Weed 1969] Weed LL. *Medical Records, Medical Education and Patient Care*. Chicago: Year Book Med Publ, 1969

[Weed 1991] Weed LL. *Knowledge coupling. New premises and new tools for medical care and education*. New York: Springer-Verlag, 1991.

[Weinstein 1980] Weinstein MC and Fineberg HV. *Clinical Decision Analysis*. WB Saunders Company, 1980.

[Whiting-O'Keefe 1988] Whiting-O'Keefe QE, Whiting A, and Henker J. The Stor clinical information system. *MD Computing* 1988; 5(5): 8–21.

[WHO 1992] World Health Organization. *ICD-10 — International Statistical Classification of Diseases and Related Health Problems*. Tenth Revision. Geneva: WHO, 1992.

[Willems 1991] Willems JL, Abreu-Lima C, Arnaud P, van Bemmel JH, Brohet C, Degani R, Denis B, Gehring J, Graham I, van Herpen G, et al. The diagnostic performance of computer programs for the interpretation of electrocardiograms. *N Engl J Med* 1991; 325: 1767–73.

[Winston 1992] Winston PH. *Artificial Intelligence*. Third Edition. Reading, Massachusetts: Addison-Wesley, 1992.

[WMA 1985] *Statement on the Use of Computers in Medicine. Handbook of Declarations*. World Medical Association. S.1., 1985.

[WONCA 1998] *ICPC-2: International Classification of Primary Care. Second Edition*. World Organization of National Colleges, Academies and Academic Associations of General Practitioners/Family Physicians (WONCA). Oxford: Oxford University Press, 1998.

[Woolf 1990] Woolf SH and Kamerow DB. Testing for uncommon conditions. The heroic search for positive test results. *Arch Intern Med* 1990; 150: 2451–8.

[Young 1982] Young WW, Swinkola RB, Zorn DM. The measurement of hospital case mix. *Med Care* 1982; 20: 501–12.

[Young 1994] Young WW, Kohler S, Kowalski J. PMC patient severity scale: derivation and validation. *Health Serv Res.* 1994; 29: 367–90.

[Zweigenbaum 1995] Zweigenbaum P, Bachimont B, Bouaud J, Charlet J, and Boisvieux JF. A multi-lingual architecture for building a normalised conceptual representation for medical language. *Proc Annu Symp Comput Appl Med Care* (19th SCAMC) 1995: pp. 357–61.

Glossary

Agent. Program that acts independently and intelligently (intelligent agent) to carry out a precise action. Agents are used on the World Wide Web to find information or to automatically index information.

ANSI. (American National Standards Institute). Organization that develops industrial standards, in particular recommendations for languages such as COBOL, C, or FORTRAN.

API. (Application Program Interface). Software that provides a set of functions and resources to provide easy access to an application program.

Applet. Small application that performs a specific task. JAVA applets make Web pages more interactive and dynamic.

ASCII. (American Standard Code for Information Interchange). International seven-bit code for representing characters (ISO-7 code).

Authoring system. Specialized, high-level language used for developing educational software that requires less programming knowledge than traditional programming languages.

Backup. Copy of programs or data files made as a safeguard against failures (hardware or software). These backup files may be restored without losing any information.

BASIC. (Beginner's All-purpose Symbolic Instruction Code). Interpreted programming language developed in 1965. Known for its simplicity.

Baud. Number of times that a data transmission channel changes state per second. In practice, a 9,600 baud modem transmits approximately 960 characters or symbols per second.

Benchmark. Standardized measure used to test the performance of various types of equipment.

Bit. (Binary Digit). The smallest unit a computer can process. A bit can have a value of 0 or 1.

Bitmap. A pattern of bits in memory that correspond to pixels to be displayed in an image on the screen. See bitmapped font.

Bitmapped font. A font where characters are made up of a matrix of points (pixels).

Bps. (Bits per second). Unit of transmission speed.

Bus. Set of conductors that transfer information between different parts of a computer.

Byte. Unit of information, made up of 8 bits.

C. Programming language developed in 1972 by Dennis Ritchie and Brian Kernighan of AT&T - Bell Labs the development of which is closely related to the UNIX operating system.

C++. Object-oriented extension of the C language, developed by Bjarne Stroustrup of AT&T - Bell Labs.

CAD. (Computer-Aided Design).

CASE. (Computer-Aided Software Engineering). Environment to assist in software development.

CBT. (Computer-Based Training). The use of computers to help people learn.

CCITT. (Comité Consultatif International Télégraphique et Téléphonique). International organization that studies and develops recommendations concerning telecommunications. Recently renamed International Tele-communications Union (ITU).

CEN. (Comité Européen de Normalisation). European organization responsible for defining standards. Committee 251 (CEN TC251) is responsible for developing standards for information technology applied to health.

CISC. (Complex Instruction Set Computer). Describes traditional computers using an extended instruction set (often greater than 100 instructions). As opposed to RISC.

Compiler. A program that translates programs written in an advanced language (such as C, C++, or FORTRAN) into code executable by a computer. Compiled programs execute faster than interpreted programs.

CORBA. (Common Object Request Broker Architecture). An Object Management Group (OMG) specification which provides the standard interface definition between OMG-compliant objects.

Courseware. Software used in education.

CPU. (Central Processing Unit). One of the three principal components of a computer, where most operations and calculations are performed.

Data compression. A technique that reduces the number of bits required to store data. Some compression techniques are designed to lose as little information as possible.

EGA. (Enhanced Graphics Adapter). IBM color graphic format whose resolution is 640×350 pixels.

EISA. (Extended Industry Standard Architecture). High-performance bus used on certain 80386 and 80486 PCs, compatible with the ISA (Industry Standard Architecture) bus.

Ethernet. Widely used communication protocol for local area networks. Initially at 10 Mbits per second, now being extended to 100 Mbits per second. Uses a CSMA/CD protocol (Carrier Sense Multiple Access/Collision Detection).

Field. The smallest data unit in a database. Fields are grouped together to create records.

Firmware. System software stored in read-only memory.

Font. In typography, a set of data representing characters (also referred to as character set).

FORTRAN. (FORmula TRANslator). Advanced programming language, developed by IBM in the 1950s, widely used in scientific applications.

Gateway. Specialized device to link together two computer networks.

GIF. (Graphics Interchange Format). Graphics format used for bitmap images. Often used on the WWW.

HTML. (HyperText Markup Language). Page description language used on the Web.

HTTP. (HyperText Transfer Protocol). Transfer protocol for Web pages on the Internet.

Icon. A pictogram used to represent an object or a function in a graphical user interface.

Indexing. Characterization of each document in a bibliographical database, with certain terms (key words) that may be used to locate the document when performing searches.

Internet. Worldwide network of interconnected computers. Uses the TCP/IP communications protocol.

Interpreter. Program that simultaneously translates and executes a program written in an advanced programming language (such as BASIC, Java, LISP).

ISDN. (Integrated Services Digital Network). Digital networking standard for high-speed transmission of data (documents, images, sound) over specialized telephone lines.

Java. Interpreted, object-oriented programming language developed by Sun Microsystems. Derived from C++, it lets programmers write interactive pieces of code, called *applets*, that may be downloaded from the Web at the same time as HTML pages.

JPEG. (Joint Photographic Experts Group). Image compression technique. The amount of information lost depends on the level of compression.

Kilobyte. (K). 1024 bytes. See byte and megabyte.

Linux. (Linus Unix). An implementation of the Unix kernel originally written from scratch with no proprietary code.

LISP. (LISt Processing). Programming language developed in the early 1960s by John McCarthy and colleagues at the Massachusetts Institute of Technology in Boston. Widely used in artificial intelligence.

Mainframe. Large, powerful central computer.

Megabyte. (MB). 1024 kilobytes. See byte and kilobyte.

MIDI. (Musical Instrument Digital Interface). Standard communications protocol for computers and music synthesizers.

MIPS. (Million Instructions Per Second). A unit for measuring the speed of a CPU.

Modem. (MOdulator/DEModulator). Device that transforms a flow of binary data into an analog signal (modulation) and vice versa (demodulation). Lets computers exchange information over the telephone network.

MPEG. (Motion Picture Experts Group). Video image compression format. Does not store each image, only the changes from one image to the next. One minute of animation requires approximately 9 MB of disk space.

MS-DOS. (Microsoft Disk Operating System). Operating system developed by the Microsoft Corporation for the Intel family of 16 and 32-bit processors. Very widespread on IBM PC and compatible computers.

Multiplexing. Technique that simultaneously transmits several signals over a single communications line.

MUMPS. (Massachusetts General Hospital Utility Multi-Programming System). Programming language associated with an operating system and data management system specially used in medicine.

Operating system. (OS). Program that manages the internal activities of a computer and its peripherals. Supervises and controls the activities of other programs.

OSF. (Open Software Foundation). Organization of hardware manufacturers and users established to promote standards for open systems.

Outline font. Font in which the characters are described as mathematical formulas.

PBL. (Problem Based Learning). Method for learning using problems, developed at McMaster University in Canada. Starting from a selected clinical case, it addresses concepts concerning both clinical and fundamental disciplines in a coordinated manner.

PCI. (Peripheral Component Interconnect). Communications bus developed by Intel. Available on computers such as IBM PC compatibles or Apple Macintosh.

PCMCIA. (Personal Computer Memory Card International Association). Association that defines standards for personal computers. Standard defining characteristics for extension cards (such as memory cards or modems) the size of a credit card. Also known as PC Card.

PCMCIA port. Socket on a personal computer that accepts PCMCIA-compatible cards such as modems, memory cards, etc.

Pipeline. A type of processor architecture first used in supercalculators, where the arithmetic and logical unit can store several instructions for quick, simultaneous processing.

PostScript. Page description language developed by Adobe Systems Inc. used by several desktop publishing programs. PostScript printers include a PostScript interpreter to translate the page description into a printable binary image. Has become a *de facto* standard.

PROLOG. (PROgramming in LOGic). Logical programming language used in artificial intelligence.

RAM. (Random Access Memory). Memory area in a computer where information can temporarily be written and read. Also called central memory.

RISC. (Reduced Instruction Set Computer). Computer with one or several processors able to execute a limited number of instructions at high speed. As opposed to CISC.

ROM. (Read-Only Memory). Memory containing information written during the manufacturing process that physically cannot be overwritten.

Router. Hardware device that transmits signals from one network to another.

Scanner. Device that reads in images, digitizes them, and transfers them to a computer.

SCSI. (Small Computer Systems Interface). Specifications for mechanical, electrical and operational standards describing the connection of different kinds of peripherals, including hard disks, printers, tape drives, etc., to a computer.

SGML. (Standard Generalized Markup Language). A formal description language for hypertext documents.

SQL. (Structured Query Language). Language used to interrogate relational databases. This is a fourth-generation language.

TCP/IP. (Transmission Control Protocol/ Internet Protocol). Set of communications standards (protocols) for transferring data (and for error correction) from one computer to another over the Internet.

Token Ring. Networking architecture in the shape of a ring, where access to write to the network is controlled by a token that passes from station to station.

UNIX. Operating system developed by Bell Laboratories in the early 1970s, now widely used on mini-computers and workstations. Is becoming a standard.

USB. (Universal Serial Bus). A standard promoted by Intel for communication between an IBM PC and external peripherals over an inexpensive cable.

VGA. (Video Graphics Array). Color graphic format developed by IBM and now widely used on PC compatible systems. The basic resolution is 640×480 pixels in 16 colors, while extensions to the standard (Super VGA) support resolutions up to 1024×768 and 1280×1024.

Videotex. Technique for transferring text and images over the telephone network. This service, called Télétel in France, is used by Minitel terminals.

VRML. (Virtual Reality Modeling Language). Language used to represent and utilize three-dimensional objects on the Web.

WAIS. (Wide Area Information Server). UNIX server on the Internet that supports keyword searches.

Web. Short for the World Wide Web. See WWW.

Windows. Software product developed by the Microsoft Corporation that provides MS-DOS machines (IBM-PC and compatibles) a graphical user interface similar to that of the Apple Macintosh.

WWW. (World Wide Web). Hypertext system that links together documents over the Internet.

WYSIWYG. (What You See Is What You Get). Term used to describe graphics systems where the information displayed on the screen is the same as what will be printed.

X Windows. Presentation and window management standard developed by the Massachusetts Institute of Technology (MIT) in Boston. Controlled by Open group.

XML. (Extensible Markup Language). A subset of the Standard Generalized Markup Language (SGML) that is designed to make it easy to interchange structured documents over the Internet. Controlled by the World Wide Web Consortium's (W3C).

Index

Numerics
3GL 10
4GL 10

A
abduction 50
abstraction 23, 52, 126
access
   direct 4
   illegal 193
   random 4
   right 199
accuracy 37
ACR/NEMA 33, 150
action 126
   plan 21
activity indicator 184
ADAM 173
ADM 86
agent 225
   intelligent 225
aggregate 25
AHCPR (Agency for Health Care Policy and Research) 180
AI (artificial intelligence) 59, 158
AID (automatic interaction detector) 185
AIDSLINE 86
AIM (Association pour les applications de l'Informatique en Médecine) 209
algorithm 1, 156
Alltel 102
ALU 2
American
   College of Radiology (ACR) 33
   Medical Informatics Association (AMIA) 209
   National Standards Institute (ANSI) 14, 225
   Society for Testing Materials (ASTM) 14, 33
AMIA (American Medical Informatics Association) 209
analysis
   cost-benefit 183
   cost-efficiency 183
   cost-utility 183
   decision 57
   discriminant 157
   DNA 166
   functional 95
   requirement 19
   structural 94
angiography
   digital 140
ANSI (American National Standards Institute) 14, 225
APACHE 188
API (application program interface) 225
applet 31, 225, 227
application program interface (API) 225
approach
   horizontal 100
   normalized 183
   vertical 98
AR (attributable risk) 203
architecture
   centralized 14
   distributed 15, 100
Arden syntax 60

ARPANET 12
artificial language 9
ASCII 3, 225
assembly language 10
association 206
ASTM (American Society for Test-
    ing Materials) 14, 33
ATM (asynchronous transfer mode)
    14, 111
ATTENDING 154
attributable risk (AR) 203
attribute 24
authentication 5, 198
authoring system 225
AZ-VUB 103

B
backup 225
base
    factual 158
    information 86
    knowledge 86, 158
baseline risk 203
BASIC 10, 172, 225, 227
baud 225
Bayes' formula 54, 202
benchmark 225
BIAM 87
bias
    cognitive 53
    judgment 53
binary
    language 9
    variable 36
biology
    molecular 87
BIOSIS 86
BISANCE 166
bit 2, 225
bitmap 225
bitmapped font 8, 225
bits per second (bps) 226
block 4
boolean
    variable 36
bps (bits per second) 226

broadcast networks 12
browser 31
    Internet Explorer 31
    Netscape 82, 211
bus 2, 226
byte 2, 226

C
C 10, 226
C++ 10, 226
CAD (computer-aided design) 226
CADUCEUS 163
card
    individual health 129
    smart 111, 198
care
    managed 108
cartography of genome 87
CASE (computer-aided software
    engineering) 226
case mix 187
CAT (computerized axial tomogra-
    phy) 140
catalog 66
    Internet 211
    of medical treatments 73
category 26
causal imputation 51
CBE (computer-based education)
    169
CBT (computer-based training) 226
CBX (computer based examination)
    174
CCITT 13, 226
CDAM 73
CD-audio 5
CD-I 5
CD-ROM 5, 86
CEN 14, 226
CEN/TC251 14
center
    activity 184
    responsibility 184
central processing unit (CPU) 2
centralized system 14
CF (credibility factor) 60

chaining
    backward 60
    forward 61
    forward and backward 63
CHIN (community health informa-
    tion network) 109
circuit
    virtual transmission 14
CISC 9, 226
classification 66
    DRG 186
    International Classification of
        Diseases (ICD) 68
    monoaxial 66
    multiaxial 67
    of nursing diagnoses 71
client-server 100
clinical practice guideline (CPG)
    212
Clinical Terms (see Read Codes)
    114
CNIL 196
COBOL 10
COCHRANE 56, 212
code
    LOINC 73
    of medical ethics 195, 196
    of public health 195
    penal 195
    Read 114
codifying 66
coding
    intensity 143
    RGB 143
    spatial 142
    temporal 143
command language 10
community health information net-
    work (CHIN) 109
commutation 206
compiler 10, 226
completeness 79
compound proposition 205
computer
    aided design (CAD) 226
    aided software engineering

(CASE) 226
    based education 169
    CISC-based 9
    handheld 6
    mainframe 6
    mini 6
    network 6
    notebook 6
    portable 6
    RISC-based 9
    virus 15, 194
computerized
    axial tomography (CAT) 140
    severity index (CSI) 187, 188
conceptual level 28
conjunction 205
connectionist system 159
connector 67, 205, 206
consensus conference 183
conservatism 54
consultant system 154
context 125
contradiction 206
contrast 143
control 180
    of therapeutic prescriptions 165
    unit 2
CORBA (Common Object Request
    Broker Architecture) 226
cost 44
    average 183
    direct 183
    estimation 102
    financial 44
    fixed 183
    health 44
    indirect 183
    marginal 183
    structural 183
COSTAR 78
courseware 171, 226
CPG (clinical practice guideline)
    212
CPT (current procedural terminol-
    ogy) 72, 78
CPU (central processing unit) 1, 2

226
credibility 54
    factor (CF) 60
CSI (computerized severity index)
    188
current procedural terminology
    (CPT) 72, 78
cyberspace 13

D
DARPA 14
data 23
    compression 226
    dictionary 33
    encryption 199
    glove 149
    integrity 194
    processing 2
    protection 194
    reliability 54
    structure 24
    type 36
database management system 28,
    126
    object-oriented 30, 127
    relational 30
DBMS (database management sys-
    tem) 28
De Morgan's theorem 206
decision
    analysis 54
    making 49
    node 57
    tree 57
deduction 49
descriptor 76
design 20
    detailed 21
    preliminary 20
development 20, 21
diagnosis related group (DRG) 180,
    185
diagnostic
    error 44
    judgment 39
    strategy 46

test 42
    value 45
DICOM 33, 150
dictionary 65
    data 33
Diogène 103
direct
    access memory 4
    manipulation 10
discriminatory value 41
disease staging (DS) 188
disjunction 205
disk
    digital versatile (DVD) 5
    magnetic 4
    optical 4
diskette 5
display screen 8
distributed system 12
distribution 206
document
    management system 83
    mediation 82
DOS 7
DRG (diagnosis related group) 107,
    180, 185, 188
drug
    contra-indication 155
    side-effect 192
DS (disease staging) 188
DSM-IV 78
duality 206
DVD (digital versatile disk) 5, 86
DXPLAIN 78

E
ECG (electrocardiogram) 132, 135,
    136
EDI (electronic data interchange)
    33, 111
EDIFACT 33
education
    computer-based 169
    permanent 114
EEG (electroencephalogram) 131,
    135

EEPROM (electrically erasable programmable read-only memory) 5
effectiveness 182
efficiency 182, 185
EFMI (European Federation for Medical Informatics) 209
EGA (enhanced graphics adapter) 226
EISA (extended industry standard architecture) 227
electrocardiogram (ECG) 132, 135, 136
electroencephalogram (EEG) 131, 135
electromyogram (EMG) 134
electronic
    data interchange (EDI) 33, 111
    mail (E-mail) 6, 11, 16
elementary
    data item 24
    data structure 24
    proposition 205
E-mail (electronic mail) 6, 11, 16
EMBASE (Excerpta Medica database) 85
EMBL (European Molecular Biology Laboratory) 166
EMG (electromyogram) 134
encryption
    data 199
endowment
    global 179
engineering
    genetic 165
    software 26
EPROM 5
equivalence 206
error
    diagnostic 44
Ethernet 12, 227
European
    Federation for Medical Informatics (EFMI) 209
    Molecular Biology Laboratory (EMBL) 166
evaluation 180

costs 182
decision support system 161
health-care 181
medical practice 181
evidence-based medicine 180
existential quantifier 207
expenses
    operating 183
expert
    system 59, 158
explanatory approach 184
external level 28

F
factor
    credibility 60
    risk 202
false
    negative 40
    positive 40
field 227
filtering
    digital 134
firmware 227
First Data 102
first-order logic 207
font 225, 227
    bitmap 225
    bitmapped 8
    outline 8, 228
formal language 205
formula 205
    Bayes' 54
FORTRAN 10, 227
fourth-generation language 10
frame 30, 60
frequency
    sampling 132
full-text
    database 83
    retrieval 85
function 207
functional unit 184

G
gateway 227

GenBank 88, 166, 212
gene sequencing 166
general contractor 21
generalist 112
GIF (graphic interchange format) 227
gigabyte (GB) 3
gold standard 40, 161
group
    diagnosis related (DRG) 180
    discussion 16
    project 21
    user 21
groupware 11, 16, 111
guideline 180
GUIDON 177

H
handheld computer 6
HBOC 102
HCFA (Health Care Financing Administration) 69, 72, 106, 180
HCPCS (Health Care Common Procedure Coding System) 72
HCUG 103
health
    information system 109
    system 106
health card
    professional 111
health maintenance organisation (HMO) 108
health-care
    cost 106
    coverage 106
    network 110
HeartLab 174
HELP 99, 164, 176
hierarchy
    is-a 76
    part-of 76
high-level vision 144
HIS
    centralized 98
    component 96
    distributed 100

HIS (hospital information system) 91
histogram 145
HL7 (Health Level 7) 33
HMO (Health Maintenance Organization) 108
holography 149
hospital information system (HIS) 91
HSTAT 212
HTML (hypertext markup language) 31, 173, 227
HTTP (hypertext transfer protocol) 31, 227
HyperCard 31
hypermedia 31, 173
hypertext 31, 173
    markup language (HTML) 227
    transfer protocol (HTTP) 31, 227

I
IBM PC 3
ICBE (intelligent computer-based education) 177
ICD-10 69, 74, 122
ICD-9 68
icon 227
ICPC-2 (International Classification of Health Process in Primary Care) 113
identification 5, 198
    of users 198
identity 206
IEEE (Institute of Electrical and Electronics Engineers) 14
ILIAD 175
image
    digitized 140
    interpretation 147
    preprocessing 145
    processing 139
    quantification 148
    segmentation 146
imaging
    scintigraphic 142

IMIA (International Medical Informatics Association) 210
implementation 20, 21
implication 205, 206
imputation
    causal 51
incidence 202
inconsistency 54
index
    relative cost 73
    severity 187
INDEX MEDICUS 76, 77
indexing 82, 227
indicator
    activity 184
    production 185
    resource 184
induction 50
inference
    engine 158
    rule 205
informatics 1
information 1, 23
    personal 196
    superhighway 13
inheritance
    multiple 30
    simple 30
input 2
Institute
    for Scientific Information (ISI) 86
    of Electrical and Electronics Engineers (IEEE) 14
integrated services digital network (ISDN) 111
integrity 194
intelligence
    artificial 59, 158
intelligent terminal 6
interaction
    between drugs 87, 165
interconnection 13
interface
    management system 127
    man-machine 10

user 161
internal level 28
International
    Classification of Health Process in Primary Care (ICPC-2) 113
    Medical Informatics Association (IMIA) 210
    Standard Organization (ISO) 13
    Telecommunications Union (ITU) 226
Internet 17, 31, 82, 115, 173, 193, 200, 227
INTERNIST 163
interoperability 102
interpretation 145
interpreter 10, 23, 227
Intranet 17
intuition 159
ISDN (integrated services digital network) 82, 111, 227
ISI (Institute for Scientific Information) 86
ISO (International Standard Organization) 13
ISO 9660 5
ITU (International Telecommunications Union) 226

J
Java 10, 31, 227
JCAHO (Joint Comission on the Accreditation of Hospital Organizations) 180
journal
    Web-based 85
JPEG (Joint Photographic Experts Group) 143, 227
judgment
    medical 53
justifiability 54

K
key word 227
kilobyte (K) 3, 228
knowledge 23, 59

academic 155
acquisition 161
causal 59
coupling 176
empirical 59
experience 155
physiological 59
representation 161
testing 173

L
LAN (local area network) 12
language
    artificial 83
    assembly 10
    authoring 172
    extensible markup (XML) 31, 33
    formal 205
    fourth-generation 10
    hypertext markup (HTML) 31
    machine 9
    medical 65
    object query (OQL) 30
    processing tools 32
    programming 1
    standard generalized markup
        (SGML) 31, 229, 230
    third-generation 10
law on computers, files and freedom
    195
learning 63
light pen 8
likelihood 201
    ratio 42
Linux 9, 228
LISP 10, 227, 228
local area network (LAN) 12
logic
    first-order 207
    predicate 207
    propositional 205
logical consequence 206
LOINC (Logical Observation Identi-
    fiers, Names and Codes) 73

M
machine language 9
magnetic
    hard disk 5
    resonance imaging 140
mainframe 6, 228
maintenance 20, 21
managed care 108
management
    committee 21
    information 1
man-machine interface 10
MB (megabyte) 228
mediation
    document 82
medical
    decision support system 153
    logic module (MLM) 60
    privacy 198
    reasoning 49
    unit 189
medicine
    curative 154
    predictive 154
    preventive 154
MEDINFO 210
Medis Groups 188
Meditech 102
MEDLARS 84
MEDLINE 77, 212
megabyte (MB) 3, 228
memory
    cache 4
    card 5
    central 4
    mass 4
    random access 4
    virtual 9
menu system 10
MERISE 20
MeSH (Medical Subject Headings)
    76, 84, 122
message 30, 33, 66
metaknowledge 159
metathesaurus 78
method

explanatory 184
MERISE 20
RACINES 21
spiral 22
methodology 19
MIB (medical information bus) 136
microcomputer 6
portable 6
microprocessor 5
middleware 102
MIDI (musical instrument digital interface) 228
minicomputer 6
Minitel 6, 230
Mips 228
MLM (medical logic module) 60
model 23
conceptual 23
hierarchical 28
mathematical 156
network 28
object-oriented 30
pharmacokinetic 162
pragmatic 125
relational 30
semantic 30
spiral 22
waterfall 19
modem 12, 228
modus
ponens 50, 207
tollens 207
molecular biology 165
monoprogramming 7
Mosaic 211
Motif 32
mouse 8
MPEG (Motion Picture Expert Group) 143, 228
MRI (magnetic resonance imaging) 140
MS-DOS 228
multimedia 1, 4, 31
server 82
workstation 16, 101
multiplexing 228

multiprocessing 7
MUMPS 10, 228
MYCIN 59, 154, 159, 177

N
NANDA (North American Nursing Diagnosis Assocation) 71
National
Biomedical Research Foundation (NBRF) 166
Center for Biotechnology Information (NCBI) 85
Center for Health Statistics (NCHS) 69, 70
Electrical Manufacturers Association (NEMA) 33
Library of Medicine (NLM) 84, 212
natural
language processing (NLP) 32, 78, 127
NBRF (National Biomedical Research Foundation) 166
NC (network computer) 6
NCBI (National Center for Biotechnology Information) 85
NCHS (National Center for Health Statistics) 69, 70
negation 206
double 206
negative
true 40
NEMA (National Electrical Manufacturers Association) 33
NEOMYCIN 177
Netscape 82, 211
network
community health information (CHIN) 109
computer 6
health 93
Internet 17
Intranet 17
local area 12
neural 156, 160
of networks 16

point-to-point 12
satellite distribution 13
semantic 25, 78
token ring 12
wide area 12
NLM (National Library of Medicine) 84, 212
NLP (natural language processing) 32, 78, 127
NNT (number needed to treat) 56
node
  contingency 57
  decision 57
noise 84, 134, 140, 145
nomenclature 65
nonambiguity 79
nonredundency 79
normalized approach 183
notebook 6
notepad 6
number needed to treat (NNT) 203

O
object 24
  multimedia 1
  selection 8
  structured 60
Object Management Group (OMG) 30
observation 126
ODBMS (object-oriented database management system) 30
odds 202
  ratio 56, 203
OMG (Object Management Group) 30
ONCOCIN 164
OODBMS (object-oriented database management system) 127
OPCS-4 (Office of Population Censuses and Surveys Classification of Surgical Operations and Procedures, 4th revision) 71
Open
  Group 230
  Software Foundation (OSF) 228

System Interconnection (OSI) 13
open system 100
operating system (OS) 8, 228
opportunity study 21
optical fiber 12
OQL (object query language) 30
OS (operating system) 8, 228
OSF (Open Software Foundation) 228
OSI (Open System Interconnection) 13
Osiris 151
outline
  font 8, 228
  isolation 146
output 2
  voice 8

P
PACS 150
Pascal 10, 172
pathognomonic 42
patient
  information system 95
  management categories (PMCs) 188
  management category (PMC) 188
  record 95, 117
pattern recognition 147
PBL (problem based learning) 228
PC (personal computer) 6
PC card 229
PCI (peripheral component interconnect)) 228
PCMCIA 229
  port 229
PCR (polymerase chain reaction) 166
PCS 98
PDA (personal digital assistant) 6
PDQ 78, 87
penal code 195
peripheral 2
personal

assistant 16
  computer 6
  information 196
PET (positron emission tomography)
  140
pharmacokinetics 156
pipeline 229
pixel 8, 143, 225
PLATO 172
PMC (patient management category)
  188
PMCs (patient management categories) 188
PMSI 73, 180, 189
point-to-point network 12
polysemy 65
positive
  true 40
positron emission tomography (PET)
  140
PostScript 229
pragmatics 34
precision 37, 84
  rate 84
predicate 208
  logic 207
predictive value
  negative (NPV) 45
  positive (PPV) 45
prevalence 42
printer 8
probability 50, 201
  a posteriori 55, 157
  a priori 55, 157, 202
  conditional 157, 201
  theory 54
processing
  data 2
  image 139
  signal 131
  word 11
processor 1
product 183
production
  indicator 185
  rule 59

productivity 27
professional
  ethics 194
  health card 111
  secrecy 195
profile
  user 199
program 1
programmed training 172
project
  group 21
  management 19
PROLOG 208, 229
properties
  behavioral 23
  structural 23
proposition 205
  compound 205
  elementary 205
propositional logic 205
protection
  data 194
  of files 198
protocol 13, 120
PubMed 86

Q
QMR (Quick Medical Reference)
  78, 163
qualitative variable 36
quality 181
  assessment 182
  assurance 181, 191
  control 180
  health-care 181
  of life 191
quantifier 207
  existential 207
  universal 207
quantitative variable 36
question
  multiple-choice 173
  true-false 173
quick prototyping 22

R
RACINES 21
radiography
    digital 140
RAM (random access memory) 4,
    229
rate
    precision 84
    recall 83
    reimbursement 106
    true negative (TNR) 42
    true positive (TPR) 42
ratio
    likelihood 42
    odds 203
    signal-to-noise 134
RDBMS (relational database man-
    agement system) 30
RDRG (refined DRG) 188
Read codes 71, 114, 122
reasoning
    abductive 50
    causal 51
    deductive 49
    heuristic 159
    inductive 50
    symbolic 58
recall rate 83
receiver 66
    operating characteristic (ROC)
        43
reception 21
recognition
    pattern 135, 147
    voice 7
record 25
    medical 197
    patient 95, 117
register 4
regression
    multiple 157
reimbursement rate 106
relation 30
relational
    database management system
        (RDBMS) 30

relationship
    explicit 80
relative risk (RR) 56, 203
reliability
    data 54
remote surveillance 111
requirement analysis 19
resolution
    contrast 143
    spatial 143
    temporal 143
resource
    indicator 184
    utilization 182
RISC (reduced instruction set com-
    puter) 9, 229
risk
    attributable 203
    baseline 56, 203
    reduction 56
    relative 56, 203
ROC (receiver operating character-
    istic) 43
ROM (read-only memory) 8, 229
router 14, 229
RR (relative risk) 56
RRR (relative risk reduction) 56
RSS 189
rule
    inference 205
    production 59
RUM 189, 190

S
SCAMC 210
scanner 150, 229
scanning 7
scenarios 21
scintigraph 146
screen 8
SCSI (small computer systems
    interface) 229
secrecy
    professional 195
security 194
SEE (software engineering environ-

ment) 26
segmentation 146
semantics 34, 205
semiology 35
    quantitative 39
sensitivity 42, 47
sequencing 166
server 15
    multimedia 82
SGML (standard generalized markup language) 31, 229, 230
sign 39
    pathognomonic 42
signal
    enhancement 134
    processing 131, 133
signal-to-noise ratio 134
silence 83
simulation 149
SmallTalk 10
smart card 5, 16, 111, 129, 198
SMS 102
SNOMED 73, 122
    RT 75
SNOP 73
software
    component 15
    engineering 26
        environment 26
    statistical 11
specialization 26
specification 20
    detailed functional 21
specificity 42, 47
spiral method 22
spreadsheet 11
SQL (structured query language) 229
standard 13
    de facto 13
    de jure 13
    gold 40, 161
    Motif 32
standardizing 121
statistical
    method 156

statistical software 11
STORM 125, 126
strategic plan 20
strategy
    data-oriented 61
    goal-oriented 61
structure
    coordinated health-care 109
    data 24
structuring 122
Super VGA 230
surveillance
    remote 111, 132
synonym 65
synonymy 65
syntax 34, 205
    Arden 60
system
    active 155
    administrator 200
    alarm 155
    authoring 225
    automatic reminder 155
    centralized 14
    connectionist 159
    critical 154
    decentralized 12
    departmental 100
    distributed 12
    expert 158, 161
    health 106
    hospital information 91
    menu 10
    open 100
    operating 8, 228
    patient information 95
    probability-based 157
    reminder 155
    semiactive 155
    watchdog 155

T
tautology 206
TCP/IP 14, 229
TDS 99
teleconsultation 110

teleconsulting 16
telecytopathology 140
tele-education 110
tele-expertise 110, 150
telemedicine 110
telepathology 110
teleradiology 110, 140
telesurveillance 111
Télétel 230
teletransmission 132
teleworking 16
theorem
    Bayes' 202
    De Morgan's 206
therapeutical trial 212
THERIAQUE 87
thesaurus 65
third-generation language 10
threshold 40
TIME 175
time-sharing 7
TNR (true negative rate) 42
token ring 12, 229
tomodensitometry 139
tomography 139
TOXLINE 86
TOXNET 87
TPR (true positive rate) 42
trackball 8
training
    at home 115
    computer-based 226
    programmed 172
    tutorial 172
transaction log 200
transcoding 80
transducer 132
tree
    AND/OR 61, 62
    decision 57
true
    negative (TN) 40
    negative rate (TNR) 42
    positive 40
    positive rate (TPR) 42
truth

table 206
    value 207
tuple 30
tutorial
    training 172
type
    data 36
    of error 45

U
UIMS (user interface management
    system) 127
ultrasound 141
    scan 141
UMLS 67, 78, 88, 122
uncertainty 53, 159
uniform resource locator (URL) 31
unit
    arithmetic and logical 2
    central processing 1
    control 2
    functional 184
    health-care 96
    visual display 8
universal quantifier 207
UNIX 9, 230
    Linux 228
URL (uniform resource locator) 31
usage right 199
USB (universal serial bus) 230
user
    category 199
    group 21
    interface 161
        management system (UIMS)
            127
    profile 199
utility 57, 185

V
validation 20
value
    diagnostic 39, 45
    discriminatory 41
    negative predictive (NPV) 45
    positive predictive (PPV) 45

truth 207
variability 36
   analytic 36
   inter-individual 37
   inter-observer 36
   intra-individual 37
   intra-observer 36
variable 207
   binary 36
   boolean 36
   dependent 184
   independent 184
   qualitative 36
   quantitative 36
VDU (visual display unit) 8
versatile disk
   digital (DVD) 5
version 22
VGA (video graphics array) 230
video sequence 171
videoconference 16, 111
videophone 16
videotex 115, 230
view 28
virtual
   company 16
   enterprise 110
   memory 9
   reality 139
      modeling language (VRML) 31, 230
virus
   computer 15, 194
visual display unit (VDU) 8
voice
   output 8
   recognition 7, 8
voxel 143
VRML (virtual reality modeling language) 31, 230

W
WAIS (wide area information server 230
waiting time 93
WAN (wide area network) 12
watchdog system 155
waterfall model 19
Web 31, 230
WHO (World Health Organization) 67, 122
wide area network (WAN) 12
Windows 7, 230
   NT 7
   X 230
WMA (World Medical Association) 194
WMRM 5
WONCA 114
word 3
   processing 11
workstation 6, 150
   multimedia 16, 101
World
   Health Organization (WHO) 67
   Medical Association (WMA) 194
World-Wide Web (WWW) 31, 230
WORM 5
WWW (World-Wide Web) 31, 230
WYSIWYG 230

X
X Windows 32, 230
X.25 14
X.400 protocol 14
XML (extensible markup language) 31, 33

Health Informatics Series
(formerly Computers in Health Care)

Transforming Health Care Through Information
Case Studies
N.M. Lorenzi, R.T. Riley, M.J. Ball, and J.V. Douglas

Trauma Informatics
K.I. Maull and J.S. Augenstein

Filmless Radiology
E.L. Siegel and R.M. Kolodner

Knowledge Coupling
New Premises and New Tools for Medical Care and Education
L.L. Weed